Please note:

Every effort has been made throughout this book [to ensure the information]
within is accurate and correct. Therefore, neither [the author nor publisher can]
be held responsible for any injury or harm resulting from [following the]
advice from this book.

Before embarking on any kind of exercise programme, it is strongly recommended that you seek advice from your GP to ensure you are ready to begin exercising.

Contents

Acknowledgements & Introduction   p05

Chapter 1
Getting started in the fitness industry   p08

Roles and titles of the instructor   p08
Get yourself qualified   p09
Register of Exercise Professionals (REPs)   p12
Code of Ethical Conduct   p13
Continuing professional development (CPD)   p14
First aid training   p15
Curriculum vitae   p15
Volunteering   p17
Gym instructing   p17

Chapter 2
Starting your personal training business   p19

Service Vs product   p19
5 P's of marketing   p20
Marketing   p21
Advertising   p22
USP (unique selling point)   p25
Promoting yourself   p26
Competition   p27
Registering your business   p27
Income tax and national insurance   p28
Manage your business   p28
Employed or self employed   p29
Deciding how much to charge   p32
Cancellation policy   p33
Where will you train your clients   p34
Risk assessment   p35
Consultation   p38
Equipment   p38

Chapter 3
Communication skills   p41

Introduction   p41
Body language and mirroring   p42
Listening skills   p44
Building rapport   p45

Stage of change — p45

Chapter 4
Fitness assessment and posture analysis — p48

VARTEC — p48
Components of physical fitness — p50
Fitness testing — p55
Relevant strength — p58
Health assessment — p59
Posture analysis — p67
Spinal conditions — p68
Screening and informed consent — p70

Chapter 5
Medical conditions — p72

Diabetes Mellitus — p72
Coronary Heart Disease — p73
Obesity — p73
Arthritis — p74
Stress — p75
Anaemia — p76
Asthma — p77

Chapter 6
Fitness principles — p79

Principles of exercise — p79
Kinetic chain exercise — p80
Dose response — p82
Overtraining — p83
Delayed onset muscle soreness (DOMS) — p84
Monitoring intensity — p85

Chapter 7
Information gathering and programming — p93

Working with different client groups — p94
SMART goal setting — p99
Barriers to exercise — p103
Finding the right weight — p103
Resistance training approaches — p105
Plyometric training — p116
Training for power — p117
Cardiovascular training approaches — p118

HIT (high intensity training)	p120
Core stability	p122
Stretching	p124
Session structure	p129
Progression	p132
Evaluation	p135

Chapter 8
Nutrition   p137

Macronutrients	p137
Carbohydrates	p138
Protein	p138
Fat	p139
Vitamins and minerals	p140
Phytonutrients	p143
Food fortification	p143
Creatine	p144
Glycaemic index	p144
Water and hydration	p145
Sports drinks	p146
Salt	p147
Alcohol	p148
Basal metabolic rate (BMR)	p149
Harris Benedict equation	p150
Excess post-exercise oxygen consumption (EPOC)	p151
Fat burning during aerobic exercise	p152
Digestion	p153

Chapter 9
Bad habits in the gym   p155

Dropping weights	p155
Bad attitudes	p157
Moaning and groaning	p157
Use of phones	p159
Posing	p159
Weights belts	p160
Inappropriate use of equipment	p161

Summary and close   p163

References   P164

Index   p165

Acknowledgements

Since my fitness career started I have been lucky enough to work with some great inspiring people. I have also been taught by some fantastic teachers and followed in the footsteps of inspiring mentors. It is all these people that I want to give a big thank you to for supporting, believing and encouraging me throughout my fitness career. I believe it is down to these people over my years as a teacher and personal trainer that inspired and enabled me to write this book. I thank you all for your continuing help and support, you know who you are.
I must also thank my students for the pictures taken and used for the front cover of this book; your time and agreement are very much appreciated. And thank you to the Southbank Club in Vauxhall, allowing the photo shoot to take place there.

Introduction

My mission was to write about becoming a personal trainer; and at the same time share all my experiences with you, and that is exactly what I have done. I hope you enjoy reading this book and get a really good idea of the fitness industry, about being a personal trainer and how to survive as a fitness professional.
Some parts of this book will be based on facts and sound knowledge, whilst others will be based on my own thoughts, beliefs and experience.
One thing I have learnt about being a fitness professional is that you have to get out there and make up your own mind about the fitness industry.
Some people want to hear facts and figures, take it away and come to decisions and produce answers based on what they have been told, really we should still be taking this information on board but making our own decision, do not deny what is true or fact, but merely choose you own route and produce your own answers, be unique.
Upon reading this book, you are either thinking of becoming a fitness trainer, just qualified and seeking further guidance or maybe you have been qualified for a while and want to refresh and extend your knowledge and understanding of the industry.

Whatever stage you are at, this book is designed to help give you an overview of many different aspects of the personal training business, from starting up and getting qualified, to running your business and keeping your clients. Throughout, I will share my knowledge, and give you my best advice based on my own experience, I'll share many stories with you as I do love to tell stories, and of course they are all relevant, just to give you a 'real' insight into being a fitness professional.

Being a personal trainer isn't for everyone, it is a great job most of the time, but can be challenging and difficult at others, also, it can be very difficult keeping up all that enthusiasm and motivation all of the time, and sooner or later you may experience burn out. Please don't let me put a damper on things, before you even get started, I just want to make you aware that it's not always easy. Being a full-time personal trainer is more than a full-time job, because when you aren't training clients you are either; travelling to the next client, writing programmes or doing other various administration work. So one thing to consider is although you may get paid a good hourly rate, this has to cover your down time too.

Personal training isn't an easy business, it isn't easy to do, and not just anyone can make personal training work for them, it takes hard work and effort. It is a constant profession, what I mean by that is, you'll be working even when you're not at work, so I say "you really have got to love it!"

I have been involved in the fitness industry since 1999, when I first started my training and decided to embark on a career in something that I actually enjoy doing myself, keeping fit that is. I can say I have never woken up and dreaded the thought of going to work day after day like so many people do, unhappy in their boring and mundane professions.

It all started for me when I visited my Auntie one day, she was doing exercise with her personal trainer, and it was one of those moments that made me think 'I would like to do that'! So from that moment I decided to get qualified and pursue a career in fitness. I had always been interested in fitness and participated in much physical activity, but it was that moment I decided to change my career.

I spent 7 years as a gym instructor, whilst studying to qualify as a studio instructor and personal trainer, from there, teaching classes on a regular basis and training a handful of personal training clients at their homes.

In 2006 I began tutoring and assessing on fitness courses and gained my certificate in education qualification which officially allowed me to deliver and teach. Now in 2014 I am still delivering and teaching fitness related courses, and passing on my knowledge and experience to people just starting out in the fitness industry.

Chapter 1

Getting started in the fitness industry

Roles and titles of the instructor

Throughout this book I will use different names to describe an Instructor involved in the fitness industry, so I thought it would be helpful to give you a brief explanation of what these roles generally are and what they entail, and perhaps you'll see something you like and want to look further into.

Fitness/Gym Instructor – writes gym programme cards, carries out gym inductions, generally advises people in the gym.
Based on qualifications, a gym instructor may carry out fitness assessments as part of the gym induction process.
This is a level 2 qualification. A level one qualification does exist, it is a gym instructor assistant, therefore not many training providers offer this; anyway, I have never heard anyone say they wanted to be an assistant gym instructor so there is no real call for it. Becoming a gym instructor is an entry level qualification; this means if you want to get started in the fitness industry, this is one of the ways in which to get started. There are other entry level courses, but which one you go for really depends on what route you want to take in the fitness industry. Sometimes a gym instructor may be asked to delivered gym-based circuits, officially a circuit training qualification is required, however, circuits in a gym is a common role that gym instructors undertake.

Personal Trainer – A personal trainer will train clients on a regular basis, in and out of the gym environment, works closely with a client to help achieve their goals.
A personal trainer will carry out fitness assessments and may also give nutritional advice for weight management; this will depend on the level of qualification they hold.
In order for you to officially call yourself a personal trainer, you need to have completed a level 3 qualification, and this will involve

an advanced training module. This is similar to the level 2 gym instructor qualification, but a deeper underpinning knowledge is required and you are also required to understand and deliver/teach advanced teaching skills and training approaches. Different training providers have different routes and time scales to becoming a personal trainer, so you definitely need to check and decide, which way is the best way for you.

Studio Instructor – Delivers group classes in a hall or studio. For example; exercise to music (aerobics), step aerobics, Zumba and circuits. Usually music is used to help structure, help participation and keep everyone in sync. Classes such as circuits sometimes use music but this will be for motivational purposes only. Studio instructors are unable to work in a gym as a gym instructor unless they possess the appropriate qualification, and likewise, a gym instructor is unable to deliver exercise to music classes. Most people who wish to teach groups exercise to music will enrol on the Studio Instructor course; this is also an entry level qualification in which further courses can be taken from.

Fitness Professional – This is the name generally given to someone involved in the fitness industry that encourages and delivers exercise and health. It is a very broad term used to describe anyone that is involved in the fitness industry.
Fitness Trainer – Another name given for a personal trainer, but could also be used to describe a fitness instructor.

Unfortunately, none of these names are legally bound, which means anyone can use them, even if they are not qualified. This obviously puts the public at risk by being trained by people who haven't been through the formal training which is needed to be suitably qualified. A company called REPs (register of fitness professionals) has been put together to safeguard the public from such trainers and to ensure they are qualified to deliver the services they offer. I will discuss REPs throughout and in more detail.

Get yourself qualified

So if you are not qualified at the moment and are just planning your training ahead to become a fitness trainer, you may be thinking what you need to do first. I suggest that you decide what kind of learning format would suit you best, different training providers will offer different delivery formats, you can complete courses over very short and intensive time periods and some over a longer period such as weekends, face to face and also home study, however, for some of the modules you need to complete during your learning will require you to attend for some face to face learning. Practical assessments are a must for qualifying as a fitness professional, as its fine just knowing what you need to do, but can you actually do it?

You will need to learn about anatomy and physiology as a fitness trainer, this is what is known as the underpinning knowledge you need to have in order to be a fitness trainer. All training providers will require you to have this, and this is the side of your qualification which helps to build your professionalism and commitment to delivering exercise.

During your learning and quest to become a fitness trainer there is much theory knowledge to learn, and at times you may think and wonder why you are learning it and how it may relate to the actual job that you are going to be doing. Well the truth is, is that much of the theory knowledge you learn won't actually be used or passed over to your clients. Please understand that I am not suggesting for a moment that you really don't need to know it, because you do, this is what makes you professional, having the 'underpinning knowledge'. So you may not pass this information you learn to your clients directly, but you will definitely use it indirectly. You see, the personal trainer and fitness instructor uses this knowledge gained to ensure the exercises they are prescribing are appropriate for the person they are training, and by understanding how the body works this can be achieved. It also gives you great credit as an instructor if the client was to ask you a question regarding the body, anatomy or physiology or a common medical condition and you can relate to the question, understand what it is they are talking about and of course give them some advice or additional information.

When you begin searching for a training provider, check the awarding body they use and ensure it is REPs accredited. I cannot stress the above statement enough, for your own sake and peace of mind. The truth is that there are many fitness training providers out there just waiting to take your hard earned money from you in exchange for their training, but not all are the same, so consider speaking to already qualified instructors to get their thoughts on training providers they went with. Visiting the REPs website and checking training providers they accredit is a much easier way to do this, and then you know the company you may decide to go with will be recognised. Having a fitness qualification that isn't recognised is no fun at all, and the last thing you want is a potential employer turning you down because your qualification isn't recognised.

These days, any gym you work for will want you to be a member of REPs, and the only way to do this is by having a recognised qualification, so make sure you don't get caught out.

If you start by checking the REPs website for a training provider, then you will avoid gaining an un-credited qualification and later wishing that you had done your homework more thoroughly! But also check the awarding body; this is the company that sets the standard and content for the training provider to deliver. The awarding body will be responsible for setting the training objectives and content for many training providers. The certificates you receive for the training you undergo will show the awarding body and the company in which delivered the training.

I am unable to give you names of training providers and awarding bodies for obvious reasons, and I certainly wouldn't want to be bias towards the companies I work for. There are many training providers out there to choose from, so ensure you do your homework first. Many providers, many costs and many delivery formats.

Just one final though on this subject, if you do decide to take a slightly cheaper route by studying at home, ensure you are realistic with your learning. How long are you going to give yourself to study in preparation for your exam? Most importantly, are you able to study at home, this is a very attractive way of studying, however, it does take self discipline and motivation.

I always found that a good way of studying and revising is to write about what you have just learnt, write it out in your own words. Or perhaps try teaching what you have just learnt to someone. Just staring repeatedly over words and pictures can often become very unproductive. Keep your studying times to around 60 minutes max, the longer you spend the less information that goes in, so do it in shorter durations but more often, and this will allow your brain to absorb the information you have just learnt, making it easier to access at a later date

Face to face learning is easier as there tends to be different styles of delivery by the tutors delivering the course, they will be (should be!) qualified teachers and therefore know how to teach in different ways and styles to allow a much more effective learning experience and environment for the student.

Register of Exercise Professionals (REPs)

The register of exercise professionals was launched in 2002, and is an independent public register which is designed to recognise the qualifications of instructors. REPs play a key role in the fitness industry as they safeguard the public from unsuitably qualified instructors and personal trainers, by providing a system of regulation; this ensures that instructors meet the health and fitness industry's agreed National Occupational Standards.

The register also ensures that trainers who are on the register are suitably qualified and able to deliver what they say they can deliver. The term 'rogue traders' suddenly pops into my head! I know there are many unqualified trainers out there, I'm sure that some of them are very good at what they do, and I know by hiring these personal trainers your house is unlikely to fall down or your electrics blow up, but it is someone's health and fitness at stake here. It seems unfair that some people spend thousands of pounds to get qualified whilst others just go straight to it without ever spending a penny, and without any formal training. So for us 'qualified' instructors, REP's is a really positive thing because they can sieve out the bad from the good in effect.

The aim for REP's is to raise public awareness of this register, and mostly to those people who exercise, go to the gym or hire a personal trainer. They would encourage every single person who wishes to seek help and advice regarding fitness and health to check whether the person they are contacting and about to seek advice from is on the register, this way the consumer gets to see exactly what training their potential personal trainer has undergone, and more importantly that they are legit.

So what does it mean to the personal trainer to be on the register? Well; from an instructors point of view, not a lot really, and being on the register won't make you a better personal trainer or instructor, it won't necessarily get you more clients, but it will show your professionalism, a commitment to the code of ethics, and illustrate your belief in the register and what it stands for.

In order to remain on the register you must show evidence of training undertaken, and if the training provider is recognised by REPs the course or qualification will then contribute towards your continuing professional development. As you continue to attend more courses and gain more qualifications you will need to keep your status up to date by uploading certificates to the website. This can be viewed by potential clients, so do not delay in getting this information on the website.

Code of Ethical Conduct

As well as regulating qualifications of instructors and trainers, REPs also aim to ensure that their members who are registered should 'establish and maintain proper standards of ethical and professional conduct when providing services in fitness instruction'.

In this industry you are seen as a professional by the public, and anyone else you may be hiring you for your services.
As a fitness professional people will trust you to look after their health and fitness, they will share personal information with you and expect it to be kept confidential, they may tell you things that they haven't told anyone else and treat you like a counselor and a relationship will undoubtedly form between you and your client, and you'll become one of your clients best friends.

These are just some examples of what happens when clients see you as a professional, so therefore, and just like other professionals; there are some rules that we must obey when dealing with the public, these are known as the 'Code of Ethical Conduct', and REPs have categorised these rules into five principles, these are:

Rights – Instructors should respect the views, individuality, needs, fairness and diversity of clients.

Relationships – Healthy relationships should be nurtured between instructors and clients.

Personal Responsibilities – Instructors will conduct appropriate and professional behaviour at all times.

Professional Standards – Fitness professionals will adopt the highest standards in their work and development.

Safe Working Practice – Clients health and safety and safe exercise environments are constantly considered.

The full description of these principles and further information about REPs can be found on their website www.exerciseregister.org

CPD (continuing professional development)

Being on the register is great, you'll get a very nice credit card sized membership card, a quarterly magazine with some really interesting stories and useful information, and also your name on the online register for anybody to view.
Of course you do have to pay this service; there is an annual fee to pay, just like any membership. But just being on the register isn't good enough, you will not remain on there year after year, and the reason being for this is because REP's need to know that you are keeping up to date with new information, learning all the time and developing your skills, something we call continuing professional development. As a member and in order for you to remain a member you must continue to keep yourself up to date and build up your CPD points. I mentioned earlier about selecting a training provider that was recognised by REP's, if it is recognised, then any training that you do will earn you CPD points, and these CPD points are what you need to stay up-to-date in the industry, show your commitment to developing your knowledge and skills, and ultimately staying on the register for all to see!
If you want to find out more about the CPD points system then I

suggest you take a look at the REP's website at www.exerciseregister.org. Here you will find more detailed information regarding this.

First aid training

It is imperative that you gain a first aid qualification when dealing with and training people on a regular basis. Hopefully you'll never need it but there might just be a chance that you will, besides, as an employed member of staff you will be expected to have it and usually paid for by the company, and also as a personal trainer your insurance may be void if you fail to keep it up to date. There are many first aid courses to choose from and the one you decide to go for should be influenced by what first aid training needs you have and the degree of risk to you and the people you will be working with are at. The most common are first aid at work, appointed person and AED with life support.

First aid at work is usually a three day course, covering; understanding the role of the first aider, basic life support, assessing situations and injuries, and bandages and dressings. This three day course is suited towards people that work in higher risk areas, team/work leaders and dedicated on duty first aiders.

The appointed person course is usually for one day only and will cover cardio pulmonary resuscitation (CPR) and basic first aid techniques; this is usually a minimum first aid qualification to hold for anyone working with the public.

AED (automated external defibrillator) life support is a one day course that is designed for first aiders and non qualified first aiders, that will train and prepare you in the use of a defibrillator and life support techniques, however, it is interesting to know that you do not have to be qualified to use an AED, and if somebody needed help, you could go ahead and use such a device if a qualified first aider was not present.

Curriculum Vitae (CV)

One of the most important things to get done once you are qualified (or even before), is to put your CV together in preparation of applying for jobs. Your CV should ideally give the potential employer an idea of what you can do, are qualified in, and skills you possess, and even though you may not have much (if any) experience in teaching fitness, you will be qualified; and your employer will be interested in what you have done in the past and how this can assist you in a fitness training role.

Your CV wants to be very informative, giving the potential employer lots of information about you, and enabling them to get an idea of whether you would be suitable for a particular role, however, we need to ensure that the amount of information we include isn't too much and overwhelming. It is far too common to overload a CV with completely irrelevant information, and even if it is, you must keep it brief to ensure you don't bore your potential employer to tears before throwing it in the bin!

When writing your CV, include dates of all jobs you have had, even if they aren't relevant, showing your employer you have had no gaps between your employment will show consistency and that you're not a slacker (hopefully not!), so do include the dates in which you had different jobs. Give a brief description of what your role was in each job and identify any relevant skills.
It is important to identify what qualifications you have, this is one of the components of a CV, and employers will be very interested in seeing in what you can actually do, although sometimes people can do things very well that they haven't actually got any qualifications to do in the first place, and sometimes even better than those who do have the qualification, needless to say, you should not include something that you are not qualified in, but it would be far more beneficial to add it to your hobbies and interests; this way you can still let people know what you do and can do.

There seems to be a big debate as to whether you should include a photo on your CV, and personally, I have always included a photo. We live in a very stereotypical world, and most people would be able to tell you what a fitness instructor or personal trainer should look like. Now I'm not saying that I look particularly like a personal trainer at all, but maybe, when a potential employer sees your photo, do they make an instant judgment as to whether or not you do look like a personal trainer? And more importantly, do they want to see you in their gym? Anyway, I can't really give you the answer to this one because everybody will have a different opinion, so my advice on this one is, if you feel you want to include it, then include it!

Volunteering

When you are applying for your first fitness job, you may be lacking in some all important experience, and it is something that most employers will want you to have, however, the fact that you have just completed your training, you are actually in a better position than some instructors who have been qualified and teaching for a while. Experience is good, but also being fresh off the block has its benefits too, and employers will recognise this.

Volunteering is an excellent way of increasing your skills and gaining experience, but not every gym will be willing to allow you to do volunteering work, although it would be beneficial to both parties if they did. So if you want to volunteer, it is obvious to say, find yourself a gym that does run a volunteering scheme, and usually with volunteering schemes you receive a really good package which may include free gym membership and possibly free training.
When you receive free training, the management is likely to charge you for any training provided if you leave within a certain period of time, so if you do not wish to stay with a company, either on a volunteering or employed basis for an extended period of time, then it is important to recognise this and be prepared to pay back for any training provided.

Gym Instructing

If you decide to do some volunteering work or begin your fitness career as a gym instructor; this is a vital part of your personal development as a fitness professional, and even if you decide to qualify as a personal trainer in a record breaking time; consider beginning with some gym instructing work, either on a part time or full time basis while you begin offering personal training to clients, this will help you gain essential experience to prepare you for your future.

The level 2 gym instructor course is an entry level qualification, and this means that it is the starting point in which people enter the fitness industry, and in my experience it has equipped me with many skills that have helped me to develop in the fitness industry.

As mentioned earlier, becoming a gym instructor by gaining your level 2 gym qualification is a foundation for your new role as a fitness professional, and for any additional courses you may take, so therefore, it might seem like a good idea to build a foundation within your own personal development and spend time at this level while you gain experience and expertise.

Chapter 2

Starting your personal training business

The following section has been put together in order to identify the business aspects that need to be considered, and a professional personal trainer will ensure that his or her business is kept up to date. Depending on what modules your personal trainer course covers; you may or may not cover most of the information that follows, none the less you should find the following information helpful.

If you plan to run your personal training business in a gym, then some of the following information may prove to be useful, however, if you plan to go freelance, then all of the following information is relevant and I hope you can use it.

Service Vs product

As I'm sure you know; personal fitness training is a service we offer as personal trainers and technically not a product we sell. Being a service and not a product has its pros and cons; on the plus side, we can offer our service at the drop of a hat, and if a potential client wanted a free taster session (try before you buy), then we could deliver without delay, we can do this as much as we like (within reason) and it doesn't cost us a thing, only time, and if free taster sessions turn into new clients, then everybody is happy. A downfall of offering a service is that during quiet times we cannot 'store' sessions for a later date, and if personal training was manufactured, then we could stock up and be prepared for busy times ahead.
If a client can actually see, touch, smell and feel a product (tangible), then they are much more likely to buy, and we can offer free sessions as mentioned before, but what we don't want to do is spend hours and hours delivering free sessions, perhaps this is fine if you are doing it for the love, but we are a running a business and a

business has to make money to survive. This is where promotional videos can help you half way in demonstrating to your client what they are buying into. This is discussed in more detail in advertising.

5 P's of marketing

Product

We discussed earlier that you are selling a service, but for this exercise we use the term product (otherwise this would be 4 P's and 1 S of marketing, not cool!). Your product is personal training; however, you may well offer a number of services that complement personal training, such as exercise classes, nutritional advice and fitness testing. Have a clear list and description of the different services you offer, a bit like a menu of exercise; what it is and what it consists of, consider making this available as a hand-out or easy to find within your website or social media.

Place

You need to decide where you will do your marketing and advertising. This should be based upon the target market you are focusing on and trying to attract. If you are targeting sports people, or just people interested in sport, then sports clubs and magazines would be an ideal place to start, where as if you were targeting 'stay at home Mums', then after school clubs and Mother & baby magazines would be an appropriate place to begin.

Price

Although being your own boss means that you can play around with your fees, having a clear pricing strategy in place is really important and allows you to give very clear guidelines for pricing to potential customers. Your pricing strategy should be fair and justified, do not under-sell yourself, but at the same time do not charge a fee that is likely to offend and put people off. Charging a lesser fee may lead some people to believe the service has no value and therefore is not very good, charge too much and you simply won't get your clients.

This is a difficult area to get right and one of the most common questions asked by new personal trainers. One strategy to adopt is to find out what the local competition is charging and what they are offering.

Promotion

What kind of promotion will you use to let people know about what you do and any offers you may have available? What kind of promotions do you regularly see gyms and personal trainers offering? You need to convince people what you have is a great deal and they would be mad to miss out. The usual 'buy one get one free' is a great promotion, but not ideal for personal training, perhaps 'buy ten get one free' is more realistic and cost effective. Decide on a promotional plan that suits you and your clients best. You will not always find the right promotional plan that works well for your personal training business, so don't be dis-hearted when it doesn't, just put it down to experience and remember not to use it again.

Marketing

Applying the appropriate marketing strategy is going to be really important if you want your personal training business to get off to a good start. First, you need to establish who your target market is going to be, this simply means, what group of people are you going to approach with your personal training business offering and focusing your promotional activities and advertising to; for example, middle aged 'stay at home' Mums. The next thing to consider is the area in which you are planning to operate in, and it goes without saying that you have to ensure that it is coherent with the target market.
It would be a great waste of your time if you targeted an area that didn't have a substantial amount of potential clients. So you will need to do your research and decide whether the target market and area chosen is viable.

If you are planning to solely operate from a gym or work as an employed personal trainer, it is likely that you will have much less marketing to do for you business, and the main reason for this is that the gym will usually do most of the advertising and promotion for you, but don't walk into a gym as a freelance PT and expect the club to suddenly give you an abundance of clients, because they won't! It will be your responsibility to find your clients, and to do this you must 'walk the floor', this is a term we use to describe the walking around and talking to people in the gym, only by doing this will you begin to gain clients. You are your best marketing tool, so getting your face shown and talking to people will soon get you clients. Ensure you also look the part, dress smartly and walk with good posture, make eye contact with people and always smile.

Advertising

Whether you are planning to go it alone as a freelance personal trainer or freelance studio instructor, it is obvious to say that you must have some kind of advertising in place in order for you to get any clients. Even if at first you plan to teach or train your friends and family, at some point along the way, some kind of advertising will be necessary. The most effective form of advertising is word of mouth, this is when somebody recommends your services to someone else, this is a very powerful means of advertisinf and people like to hear first hand recommendations, especially when it comes from a friend or relative. Many personal trainers I know rely only on this kind of advertising, and technically once they gain one or two clients, they don't have to do any other advertising at all.

The use of social media like Facebook and Twitter has become very popular for fitness professionals to reach out to people about their business. It is important to realise these platforms should not be used for direct advertising with post after post and message after message about your business, this would be no different to the junk mail you receive through your door, pick up and put straight in the bin without even looking at it because you know it's rubbish, and it annoys you that people keep on posting this stuff to you! If you do use social media, open a business page and invite people to like it, give information about you and what you do. Allow people to browse and not feel like you're giving a hard sell. Potential clients do not see the idea of personal training for the first time and decide to go with it, most people follow the model below before making a buying decision.

The AIDA model suggests that people go through a series of mental stages before making a financial commitment.

Awareness

People must be aware of a product or service before going further towards making a decision, I know this is an obvious statement, but if people don't know about your business, how can you expect them to become your customer!

Interest

It is suggested that people have to be exposed to a particular product or service about seven times before they make a connection to it. At this stage, consider the effectiveness of leaflet dropping, this model suggests you would have to leaflet drop the same area of houses seven times before any of its occupants took any notice of your offering, doesn't sound like a good deal to me. So here you will need to consider ways in which to get your potential clients interested and increase their knowledge of the service you offer.

Desire

Once an interest has been established, the next stage for the purchaser will be to make the service or product desirable to them. As an example, have you ever seen a particular product or service advertised and you've thought, 'I don't really need it, but I really want it'? If the answer is yes, then you will start to justify reasons why you should have it and how it will change you, make your life easier and the way you do particular things. You may decide to impulse buy at this stage; this is usually due to the fact that you just want it, then you may experience buyers' remorse after the purchase and continue to question yourself whether or not it was the right thing to do. The best buys are achieved when the product or service purchased is actually something that the buyer truly wants or needs. So let's bring this back to personal training, and I can tell you from experience that people do not impulse buy personal training sessions before a desire has been established, and at this stage your potential client is aware of his or her health, they know about personal training and have been thinking about it for some time, they will do their research about the service, talk to other people about it and begin to see themselves actually doing it.

Action

This is when they make that call, to you, their potential personal trainer. At this stage, your client is almost fully committed to making a decision, that decision, to have a personal trainer, or at least to try it. They have been introduced to the idea, found the idea interesting, justified reasons for doing it and are ready for the next stage. So there shouldn't be any hard sell from this point, or at any point for that matter, all you have to do is convince them that you are the right personal trainer for them, should be easy if you are the right type of person to do personal training! What you should also consider here is how you allow your potential client to action their decision, how can they contact you? Ensure this part is made very clear, otherwise you may lose out, and so might your client.

There are lots of things to consider when putting together an advertising strategy for your personal training business. Below are five key areas:

- Mission. What is the mission or the aim of your advert? What is it that you wish to achieve from it? Perhaps it is to increase public awareness, highlight a promotion you have, or to inform people of an event that is happening. Whatever it is, ensure it has an aim; what exactly is the goal?

- Money. What budget do you have for your advertising? Be clear on how much you have to spend and keep the figure realistic. Many adverts can be designed yourself on computer software but may lack that professional touch, however, it will save you money. Many forms of advertising are free, particularly with social media platforms, so it is definitely worth seeking these out and taking advantage of them.

- Media. Capturing the right audience is crucial, so therefore the type of advertising you choose is also really important. You may want to place an advert in a mother and baby magazine if you are targeting post natal clients, or wear a branded t-shirt whilst floor walking in the gym. Some types of media will have huge cost implications, for example television and radio can charge extreme amounts of money, particularly during peak viewing and listening times.

- Message. What is the message that you are trying to get across to your target market? What do you want your advert to say? What do you want your target audience to think? This is where you have to spark an interest and desire for your service. Ensure the message is clear and also add different ways to respond to the advert, i.e. telephone, email etc.

- Measure. How are you going to measure the interest? And how will you know if the advert has worked? You must ask potential clients where they heard about you, this way you can identify the most effective forms of advertising. It may be worth setting yourself targets in respect of how much response you are expecting, and this will help to identify whether or not the type of advertising is appropriate.

USP (unique selling point)

More and more people are becoming qualified as personal trainers, and training providers are continuously delivering fitness courses; producing hundreds and hundreds of new fitness professionals, meaning your competition increases day by day, and that means you need to stay ahead of the game and ensure you're offering something that your competition isn't, something that will encourage people to hire you as a personal trainer and not your competitor.
Your USP can be anything that makes you stand out from the crowd, the most colourful and sharpest pencil in the pencil case maybe! It may be that you offer a unique service or product that no other trainer offers, or it may be something personal about yourself, which you think makes you stand out from the rest. Whatever it is, make sure people know about it through your marketing and promotion.

Promoting yourself

As discussed already, personal training is a service and not a product, and therefore it is difficult to put it on a shelf or advertise it online, people cannot see it until they buy it. This is a huge barrier for personal trainers as we're sure people would love to buy into personal training, only if they knew exactly what they were getting into. If you operate from a gym, then it is likely that your potential clients will seen you training another client, and they like the way you work, can see that the client is getting a great service, and they want a piece of that. If you operate outside of the gym, you might be lucky enough for people to spot and approach you in an outdoor environment, and my advice here would be for you to wear a branded t-shirt with your business name and contact details, so in case people didn't feel comfortable approaching you, they could at least take your contact details and then get in touch at a later date. Wearing a branded t-shirt when you train clients at their own home won't do much for promoting your business but it will of course make you look professional, so wear it all the time, this could then lead to your client referring you to a friend or member of the family. Also look smart and tidily dressed, ensure you have spare work t-shirts, a clean looking pair of trainers, and a suitable pair of tracksuit bottoms or shorts. These clothes are your work clothes, and just because we don't have to wear a suit to work, it doesn't mean that we can get away with looking scruffy! Keep your head and facial hair clean and tidy (men only for the facial hair!). Smell fresh; if you don't have the time to shower between sessions; then ensure you have some deodorant to spray on!

Promotional video

If you want potential clients to see what you do, then consider putting together a promotional video, this should give the viewer a clear image of what you do and how you do it. You should begin with an introduction, done personally by you is best, include snippets of you training clients (try to include a range of clients, this will help your potential client to relate to a particular group of people you train), avoid making the video about you and make it about what you can do for and can offer your client. Ensure you include plenty of

contact details in the video, so people have a range of ways to get in touch.
If you already have one or more clients, ask them to give you a video recorded testimonial, this will really boost the profile of your personal training business and is likely to boost your clientele.

Competition

One of many steps to take when venturing out on your own is to check out the competition. What are other personal trainers doing in your area doing? How much are they charging? Where are they operating? These are just a few questions that you might want to try and find out. You may not get the whole picture, but it is certainly an advantage to you if you can find this out. How might you do this? Well, one way I would suggest is to get online, and access details of trainers in your area. The REP's website (www.exerciseregister.org) and the National Register of Personal Trainers (www.nrpt.co.uk) will give you details of personal trainers within a particular area, this of course is only if they have registered themselves with these sites, and as we discussed earlier, many haven't. There are also many other personal trainer directories on the internet, so take the time to check these out too.
You may even be tempted to call some of these trainers, act as a potential client, discuss what they can offer you, find out prices, and where they operate. This may sound a little sneaky, but it may be that you want to offer something different to your competing fellow personal trainers, and in this case you are actually looking out for them. Let's face it; they're not going to just tell you everything if you expose yourself as their competition.

Registering your business with HMRC

If you are to become a self-employed trainer, it is vital that you contact HMRC to register your business and self employed status. Even if you are still in the process of gaining your qualifications, it is still worth getting in touch to let them know (www.hmrc.gov.uk). Try and set a date in which you intend to start your business as well, setting a date can help you stay focused and motivated. The HMRC website is very useful with lots of relevant information to help you get started and what you need to do.

Income tax and national insurance

As a freelance personal trainer you must pay your own income tax and national insurance based on the profit your business has made. Once you have registered with HMRC and it's time to file your self-assessment; tax and NI will be calculated automatically for you based on the information and figures you declare. Although filing your own tax return is generally thought of as a hassle, it is in fact very easy as long as you keep all your paperwork tidy and manage your business effectively (see next section). Hiring an accountant is wise if you have piles and piles of paper work to sift through your accounts and no time to do it, but it can be done yourself with ease, especially if you decide to file your return on-line. You must register for on-line self assessment and you will be given a username and password to access your account at any time.

Manage your business

By following a few simple rules, you can effectively manage your business, maintain a smooth running and keep all paperwork up to date and tidy.

- ➢ Keep a simple cash flow account, update it daily in order to stay on top of things, this can give you an accurate day to day account of profit and loss, you can either purchase a double cash book, or create an account with specific software or excel.
- ➢ Open a separate bank account for your personal training income, avoid depositing your income into your personal account, keep it separate, this will make life a whole lot easier when it comes to self assessment, besides, it's more professional.
- ➢ Keep all receipts and invoices for taxable purchases. The use

of a plastic wallet or envelope works well, this way you can separate receipts for every month or tax year.
- Give receipts and invoices to clients and ensure you keep a copy. When a client pays you money, ensure you give them a receipt, you can easily purchase receipt pads that are carbonated and therefore leave you with a copy once you have torn out your clients copy. I also like the idea of sending my clients an invoice, and I usually do this electronically, even if the client has paid me. Include information of sessions including dates and fees. By doing this you also have a back-up of the dates that you have trained your client, and which should marry up to the dates in your PT diary.
- Use a diary to keep a track of client appointments, even if you only have one or two sessions a week and you can easily remember when you are seeing them. You may want to insert how much and when they paid you, and as the sessions go on, highlight how many session or money they have left.
- Keep all bank statements related to your business, this will show additional proof of purchase of items bought. If you do not have a separate bank account, then highlight all income and expenditure with a highlighter pen.

It is very important to keep all this paperwork safe and secure for your own benefit, keep it organised and easy to find. You are bound by law to keep records of self employed income for seven years, if you are inspected and fail to show records for a particular trading period, you can be fined up to £4,000.

Employed or self-employed

One of the main decisions you will need to make when starting your personal training business is whether you want to operate within a gym, or outside of a gym, you could even do both if you wanted to, and this would be financially beneficial. So let's discuss some advantages and disadvantages to both.

So let's begin with working for a large chain gym, all gyms will operate a slightly different system for personal trainers so obviously you will need to do your research for wherever you plan to work.

Employed as a PT with fixed hours – the first benefit of being employed is that you will not have to submit a self assessment to HMRC, and your employer will deal with paying all your taxes and National Insurance, you will have set weekly hours and usually you will be expected to spend an amount of time as a gym instructor, walking the gym floor and doing regular inductions. As you may well know, you will also get holiday pay and all those kind of benefits you are entitled to as an employee of a company, but do check your contract before you sign it. You will not be frowned upon if you wish to look over your contract, rather than jump straight in and sign it when you don't know exactly what you are agreeing to.

Freelance (self-employed) PT paying monthly rent – this is a very common way in which PT's operate within a gym, although each club may vary, essentially, the idea is the same. With most large chain gyms, you are not employed, but self employed, and this simply means you have to complete and submit a self assessment to HMRC at the end of every tax year and pay any money you owe, this is a relatively easy task, especially since you have been able to submit it online. See the Tax & National Insurance section for more information on this. You will be expected to wear the club branded uniform, which will usually be a t-shirt minimum, the uniform will have the clubs logo on it and also have personal trainer or similar printed on the back, this will help other staff to identify your role within the club and also a great tool to advertise to potential clients. The club will charge you rent each month for the use of their club, and in some cases, the club will introduce a sliding scale rent fee for the first few months, this is to give you time to build up your clientele and therefore enabling you to afford your rent; you are responsible for finding new clients, and not the club, so time is precious in the first few months, and you must remain proactive if you want to find new clients.
A major issue you will face with this operation is the competition from other PT's, although it is unlikely that all personal trainers are operating from the same club 24 hours a day, you may be competing with up to as many as 20 other PT's. The problem here is; because the monthly rent will be substantial, you will be keen to work as many hours from a single venue, once the rent threshold per month has been met, then everything else is yours, see the example below.

Monthly rent = £900 per month
PT session per hour = £45

20 sessions per month = £900 (rent threshold)
60 PT sessions delivered per month = £2,700

£2,700 - £900 = £1,800

This example indicates a profit of £1,800 after the rent has been paid, once the rent threshold has been met you will feel eager to deliver as many session as possible, although you will have to pay tax on your profit, at least you know the money you are making is yours and you're not paying any more than necessary to the club.
Another way that the club may want to be paid is a percentage of what you earn, or to charge you a set fee for each session you deliver, this is an ideal way of operating if you don't want to commit yourself to a single venue, or if you only want to do a few hours a week without having to pay a high rent, however, finding a venue that allows you to pay per session may prove harder than you think.

If the idea of working in a gym for the majority of your working hours and paying someone else your hard earned money doesn't do it for you; then the other option is operating either outside or at your clients' house. Even though you will still have some financial outlay, it can be far more satisfying knowing that the money you earn for every session is going to you.
Training at your clients' house will cost you nothing, not unless your client wants to charge you rent for the use of their house! No, this is very unlikely, I have never experienced this. You do need to travel to meet your client though, this will mean you need extra time and have to spend extra money on travelling. You must consider these extra expenses when deciding on how much to charge your client, this is covered in more detail in the next section, Deciding how much to charge.

When you operate outside a gym, you are immediately faced with the issue of limited equipment. Sometimes it would be nice to have access to unlimited pieces of equipment, however, when you don't have this luxury, it does encourage you to be a lot more inventive with exercises you deliver, and it also keeps things exciting and different for the client. There is a great deal of small portable equipment on the market, and with this equipment you can deliver some amazing personal training sessions that your client is going to love, and with so much choice you are bound to find something for everyone. In my experience, not all clients are going to like all the different type of equipment you have, but if you do have a broad range then you are more likely to please everyone, and ultimately keep your clients. Later on in this section I have put together a list of equipment that is mostly portable, relatively cheap and will hopefully meet the majority of your equipment needs.

Deciding how much to charge

Deciding on what price to charge for your services is going to depend on many factors. The biggest factors will be whether you are gym based, working from a clients' home, or working outside and the area (geographic) in which you are operating. Do your market research; this will help you to establish what the competition is charging for the type of service they are offering. Charging a higher rate and delivering a lesser service isn't going to get you very far, so ensure you keep your rate reasonable and deliver a service in line with it. You would be right in thinking if you charge a higher rate your target market will take one look and walk away, that can be said for the majority of people, but for others, a higher rate means a higher quality, so some people will be attracted to that, but you must be able to justify your premium rate. On the other hand, if you charge a much lower rate, people may look at it as a reduced quality service and still be turned off by the fact. Here is the example I like to use when discussing the quality and price to charge for personal training: If you walked into a well known sports shop and saw a pair of trainers that had your name written all over them, I mean, you look at them and you instantly fall in love with them, you imagine yourself wearing them, you think about how good you feel wearing them and how good they look on you. You want them and you know you will have them. You check the price tag and they are a little pricey, but your love for them overrides the price, you decide to get them next week when you get paid. In the meantime, you see an identical pair of trainers at the local Sunday market for nearly half the price! So what do you do? Do you splash out the cash for the pair you saw in the sports shop? Or do you buy the much cheaper pair from the market? Could the quality be affected by the price of the cheaper pair? Will the most expensive pair last you longer? It's a difficult one, but this could be true for personal training too.

If you are based at one location, you may decide to charge a set fee, and that would be the sensible thing to do, however, your fee should change if you are travelling to your clients home, as the big difference here is travel time and costs. One way in which you could set your fee is by charging a flat rate, and then add on the mileage and travel time. For example, if I set my flat rate at £25, my client lives 10 miles away and it takes 30 minutes to travel there by car, all together that is 1 hour travel time and 20 miles, so here is how I would calculate it.

1 hour PT session £25 (flat rate)
1 hour travelling £10
20 miles @ 45 pence per mile £9

Total £44

Cancellation policy

Having a cancellation policy in place can and will save you much potential grief in the future, sometimes clients will let you down; intentionally and unintentionally, either way, a cancellation policy needs to be in place and highlighted at the start, introducing it at a later stage can be a little awkward, especially when you feel you should charge your client for a cancelled session. If your client gives you notice should they need to cancel, then it may be possible to fill the gap with another client who may be desperate to see you for another session, but if the client calls you just hours before, or even lets you down when you arrive at their house for the session, then you have to charge for the inconvenience caused and time wasted, all professions have a cancellation policy in place, and we are no different, you would be expected to pay for a missed dentist appointment wouldn't you?
Usually, 24 hours notice is required before a charge is made, but this is up to you, if your client is unwell, calls to cancel at the last minute

and you wouldn't have filled their space with another client, then you may decide to not charge and just rearrange the appointment/session. Whatever you decide, make your rules clear to the client from the start, and consider some kind of agreed contract between the two of you, explaining payment and cancellation, get them to sign it, and this way they won't get a surprise when they find out you've billed them for a cancelled session.

Where will you train your clients?

As a personal trainer, you have to decide where you want to train your clients, this can either be; in a gym or PT studio, at the clients house, or outside. They all have their advantages and disadvantages, and you will need to decide where you will operate your business. You will certainly need space at home in which to do your admin work, whether it is a spare room or a small area in the dining room, working as self employed, it is essential that you have somewhere to call your office, no matter how small the area is.

If you decide to operate from a gym, then you have complete use of all the equipment that the gym has to offer, this is a massive advantage, and therefore neither yourself or your client ever needs to supply or purchase their own equipment, the disadvantage is that you may become lazy when it comes to designing programmes, and encourage you to do very similar things with many clients, and therefore not making the programme specific to the individual.

Training your client at their home allows you to be very creative with your session design, and during consultation with your client (assuming the consultation takes place at their home), you will be able to identify how and what you are going to do with your client on their first training session. When assessing space and equipment availability, you must not allow this to be a barrier, instead see it as a challenge that will help develop your skills as a personal trainer that has to adapt to different situations. You will need to possess some equipment when training clients at home, that's not to say that you have to use equipment, because there are many cardiovascular and bodyweight exercises that can be done without the use of equipment, but as time passes, you will need to progress your clients programme and exercises, and without any equipment whatsoever, this may prove to be difficult.

Some clients may already have their own fitness equipment, or be keen to purchase some once they start training with you, this may save you some effort of carrying equipment around with you, hopefully this will also encourage your client to do some exercise at home themselves, but don't bank on it, many clients that I have seen in the past are not keen to exercise unless I am there with them.

The main disadvantage to training people at their home is the fact that you have to travel to and from; this then incurs time and travel implications. However, there is no rent to pay, and you can also use the expenses travelling to and from your clients' house to off-set your tax when you do your accounts and submit your tax return at the end of the year.

The outside environment offers many training possibilities when it comes to exercise, for example, hills and steps can be ideal for aerobic exercise, also if you have access to a sand or stone beach, this can reduce the amount of torque produced through the legs and up the intensity of walking and running.
Apart from bodyweight exercises that can be performed anywhere without equipment, you need to look around the environment, and use your imagination if you want to perform muscular strength and endurance exercise. Low level walls, benches, monkey bars and railings can all be used to achieve this. Cross-training in an outdoor environment can be a really effective way of training your clients, giving them a whole body workout and prevention from over-training.
When training, particularly outside, health and safety of your client, and yourself for that matter, is paramount, a thorough check of the environment and a full risk assessment should take place in order to highlight and minimise any risks involved.

Risk assessment

Before you begin teaching in any environment, you must ensure a full risk assessment has taken place, this is done to highlight any risks that may cause harm to yourself or your client, and to assess ways in which to minimise those risks. Most companies have to carry out risk assessments by law, as personal trainers we don't, however, for good customer care and everybody's safety, we should do it and take it seriously.

If you work in an outdoor environment, then you will have many areas of risk assessment to consider, let's highlight these areas:

First aid facilities

Do you have a first aid qualification? Do you have a first aid kit? Is there anyone in the surrounding vicinity that can deliver first aid if necessary? The welfare of your client should be in the forefront of your mind at all times. The first rule of being self-employed is to ensure that you have a valid first aid certificate, and if you do not have a first aid qualification, you may just end up in a sticky situation.

Many public places now have defibrillators in case of medical emergency, and everyone (qualified or not) is encouraged to use it. They are very simple to use and fully automatic, therefore it tells you exactly what to do, according to the given situation.

Toilets

One of the biggest issues when it comes to working in an outdoor environment is whether or not there are toilet facilities, and there is no more unsettling feeling than being caught out without a toilet. For most people, relieving yourself in a concealed place does not bother or concern them, but of course this is not always appropriate or convenient. So if the area in which you are planning to take your client does not have a toilet, make sure you find out the location of the nearest facilities, so if the worst does happen, at least you know of somewhere in an emergency.

Water availability

When training clients indoors, water and refreshments availability do not seem to be an issue, and these tend to be readily available. It is really important to remain hydrated throughout the session, so always encourage your client to bring water along to their session. Water in an outdoor environment is sometimes hard to come by, however, if you are close to a café or pub, most people seem happy to serve a glass of tap water if you ask nicely. If you are using your own transport, carrying spare bottles of water for your client is a really nice touch and can be a lifesaver when you really need it.

Parking facilities
Does the venue or location in which you are training have parking facilities for you and your client? Some outdoor venues may have parking restrictions, so be sure to investigate, or if they are travelling by public transport; can they get there easily. You also need to ensure that you can easily get to and from your outdoor venue, especially if you have equipment to carry around.

Lighting (after dark)
Depending on the time you will train outdoors, you may need to know for everyone's safety if there is lighting after dark. It is not suitable or ideal to be training outdoors as it starts to get dark, technique may be compromised, and being unable to see the surface in which you are training on may make things very hazardous. If you do train your clients at night and you have no way of avoiding the dark, then consider a flashlight or a head torch to take with you.

Permission
If you are planning on training your clients in the park, then you must contact the council in which the park belongs to in order to gain permission. Some councils' may not require you to pay a fee or rent, but outdoor fitness training has become very popular and most councils are recognising this, and therefore charging for your use. You may argue that 'who's going to know?' and decide to go ahead without prior permission, but it would be rather embarrassing if you are in the middle of a PT session when a park official questions you regarding a usage license! It may be that you are setting up a group fitness session, and there will be no doubt, from a park officials' point of view that you are teaching and earning money. Best to be safe than sorry.

A risk assessment should also cover aspects of the client, for example, appropriate clothing, ensuring the client has been fully screened (ParQ and questioning), any injuries, consent gained etc.

Consultation

In my experience, if you have managed to arrange a consultation with a client, then they are very likely to take you on as their personal trainer, but we shouldn't assume this for one minute, but focus on it as an opportunity for your potential client to make up their mind about you. We must make a positive impression towards our client, not only during the consultation, but consistently throughout your relationship, so make the first meeting a positive one; remember the first impressions rule?? Within the first few minutes your client will decide whether they like you or not, and you never get another chance at making a first impression, unless you have a time machine of course! The consultation has many purposes, as well as the above, you will need to find out a lot about your client if you are to write them detailed plans and deliver sessions that are very specific to them, their goals, and needs.

It will be worth considering where you will conduct your consultations with clients. If you are operating from within a gym, then obviously in the gym or maybe somewhere in the club such as the cafe would be the ideal place to do this, however, if you are training people outside of the gym, consider a public location where you can both feel relaxed, such as a coffee shop. Some people will not mind you visiting them in their home, but we also need to consider ourselves, and maybe we feel the need to meet our new client for the first time in a mutual environment.

Equipment

If you are planning on working for a gym and ultimately running your business from there; you have the luxury of all the cardiovascular and resistance equipment to choose from, and there will be no need for you to buy your own equipment. Most gyms these days have a massive selection of equipment, the only problem you may experience is when you want to use something, and somebody else is using it, and this might happen more frequently during busy times, unless it is a really large gym. I wouldn't advise it but I have seen some personal trainers use 'reserved' or 'out of order' signs on equipment, ensuring that nobody steps in at that crucial time.

As a self-employed freelance personal trainer, you are going to need to buy some equipment, and depending on where and how you operate, this will affect the amount and type of equipment you have. In my experience as a personal trainer, for the majority of my career I have visited clients in their own home and have driven there, this makes it easier to transport a selection of portable equipment. I have always liked the idea of buying a lorry and kitting it out with a treadmill and other large non-transportable equipment, but of course, an operation like that would be very expensive and in some ways not very practical. All the fitness equipment I possess I can get in my car, maybe not all at once, but depending on what my client wants to do, I can select the type of equipment I need. Even without a car, or your own transport, there is still a very large selection of equipment out there which you could fit in a back pack, be able to easily transport it, and still offer your client a workout of their choice.

Some of the equipment you buy can be very multi-functional, enabling you to use it for many different things, whilst others may only offer a single use. Below is a list of some portable equipment you might consider purchasing for your business, remember you can get tax relief from any equipment bought for your business.

Resistance bands – It is best to have a selection of these that vary in resistance to accommodate a range of clients. Although resistance bands only cover a single use, they can be used to provide a resistance workout to most areas of the body, you just need a little imagination.

Dumbbells – A good tip is to buy a set of dumbbells with removable plates, this way you can easily adjust the weight to suit different exercises, and it saves you having several sets of dumbbells to transport.

Aerobic step – This is a really versatile piece of equipment as it can be used for so many things, although it is bulky, it is relatively light. It can be used as a bench when using weights, a little lower than the type of bench you would find in the gym but it does the job. Simply stepping up and down is a great form of aerobic exercise, using it for the warm up and the main aerobic workout.

Swiss ball – A swiss ball is a great piece of equipment for strengthening the core, its unstableness works the proprioceptors in your muscles which help to improve balance and spacial awareness. It can also be used as a bench for some resistance exercises; offering a much less stable surface to work upon, making the exercise harder, and challenging the participant further.

Boxing equipment – The use of pads and gloves has become very popular with personal trainers, and many training providers now offer courses to learn basic striking techniques, using this equipment can help the client to improve all components of physical fitness.

Suspension kit – A really small, light and portable piece of equipment, allowing you to cover a whole body approach and increase muscular strength and endurance. The most well known brand that most people associate with suspension fitness is TRX, but there are many other brands to choose from. You must ensure a solid anchor point for this equipment before use.

Medicine balls – A weighted ball allows you to perform exercises with resistance that you may not find suitable to do with conventional free-weights, for example, throwing and passing, and its spherical shape makes it much easier to handle. Consider the weight of the ball you purchase to ensure it is suitable for the majority of your client group; unless you are planning to buy a whole collection!

Exercise mats – These are of course essential for your client, some clients training at home will be quite happy to lay on their carpet or grass without one, but you will need one none the less, particularly if you are outside on a cold and hard floor.

Chapter 3

Communication skills

The most important part of being a personal trainer has to be your ability to communicate with people and adapt to different client personalities. Motivation is also very important and one of the biggest reasons people want to train with a personal trainer, this may be why there is a number of trainers out there training clients who aren't actually qualified, and as I have mentioned before, the title 'personal trainer' has no legal bounding. There are obviously a number of things wrong with not being qualified, the main issue would come down to insurance and without appropriate qualifications there is no valid insurance, this is going to be like driving a car without a driving license, and also unqualified instructors are doing an injustice by lying to clients. Secondly, if the so-called personal trainer has no formal qualifications, then they may be less aware of how the body works, therefore not allowing them to prescribe safe and appropriate exercise to their clients.

Much of the time clients may just need to offload and want someone to talk to, so sometimes we end up feeling like counsellors, and that session you spent a long time designing doesn't get delivered, and somehow you feel like you're the one that has been short-changed, but at the same time feel guilty as your hourly rate that you charge your client doesn't justify the work that you have done.

As a personal trainer you need to be able to adapt, there are and will be many adaptations you will have to consider and implement. One of the adaptations you will need to make is based on the type of client you have and the relationship you have with them. I very much believe in adapting your personality to the client, I don't mean being or acting like someone different, I mean just trying to mirror their personality and ways. There is much evidence to prove that we like people who are like us, so the more we can be like our clients, the more they will like us, and the more they like us then they are more likely to continue to employ us as their personal trainer, and of course it goes without saying this means more income for us.

If there is only one thing you do to help build rapport with your clients and make them feel important, it is to call them by their name. Now I know this sounds obvious and you may be thinking; 'well I'm not going to call them by someone else's name', but, what I mean is, from day one and your first meeting with them, continue to address them by their name, this will instantly build rapport and 9 times out of 10 your client will feel an instant bond with you. Many companies employ this technique with their sales teams as they know the power of using it, and it may explain why so many people open their doors and invite sales people in to their house to sell them inappropriate products that they never ever use or need, even persuade and bully people into buying things once they have got their foot in the door (literally)! I can certainly remember a few times that this happened to my family, but we won't go into that, I'll save you the boredom and the unnecessary need to diverse from topic.

Now I'm not suggesting we bully people into buying personal training; no this would never work, what I am suggesting is that we do whatever we can to establish rapport with our clients right from the very start, this will allow our potential clients to trust us, and most importantly, buy into us.

Body language and mirroring

Let's talk for a while about body language, particularly during a consultation with your client. This has to be one of the most crucial times of the client deciding whether or not to go with you as their trainer. The fact is that they have already decided that they want personal training; that's in the shopping basket, their next decision is which checkout to go through! (Metaphorically speaking) What's really important now is that you make the right impression on them.

People like people who are like them, so try and mirror their ways, their personality, and also the way you talk to them based on their age, class and beliefs.

Mirroring is a very effective technique used to build rapport with people, and is a very clever way of achieving it without making it look like you're trying; this is because it's done silently. The thing to remember though is not to go overboard with this one, because it will appear obvious, you will be sussed straight away and you run the risk of looking like a fool. This is a skill you must develop slowly through experience, but if you remain aware of it from now on, then you can start working at it.

I am going to assume that most people know that when you are seated talking to someone (this is usually the best way to conduct a consultation with a client, I have never tried it standing up), ideally we shouldn't be directly opposite them, this can feel a little uncomfortable for the client and sometimes the trainer too, if you are in the direct line of your potential clients eyesight it can make one feel quite uncomfortable and often intimidated. Have you ever been on public transport during a really busy time when there has been standing room only? Have you ever suddenly found yourself directly face to face with someone? I have and it's not the best feeling, especially if they have bad breath, not nice at all. Luckily this doesn't happen very often, because what you will find and perhaps be aware of from now on is that people tend to turn away from each other slightly, being very close to someone isn't the issue (unless they smell for whatever reason), it's the direct line of eye contact. Try this exercise, next time you are in company, and not with someone you are intimate with, stand directly in front of them, oh be sure to tell them why and what you are doing just in case they get a little scared or concerned. You don't have to be touching noses but do make sure you're close and directly in front. Spend a short while there just enough to make a mental note of how you feel, then stand side by side and touching shoulders, see how being even closer but not in direct eyesight of your helper feels less awkward or intimidating.

Eye contact is really important when building rapport, it shows interest, confidence and lack of shyness in a person, however, do not start staring people out for long periods of time, unless you want to appear like Jack Torrance from The Shining and more importantly, lose a potential client! In my experience, approximately seventy five percent of the time is appropriate to make eye contact, and including the use of hand gestures (as you speak), can give you something else to focus on momentarily.

Listening skills

Listening skills are really important; even more so as a personal trainer, it demonstrates that we are interested in what the speaker is saying, it also helps us to understand and respond appropriately.

It may be easy to hear someone talking but are you really listening to them, and have you ever found yourself drifting away and becoming distracted while someone is talking to you, then realising you cannot recall what they were saying? This happens all too often, but I would bet that if you were to do this during your consultation with a client, they would be quick to back out. It is fair to say that some people have a natural ability to send you to sleep as they speak, especially if they remain monotone and fail to keep you engaged, but unfortunately we cannot ask our clients to speak to us with enthusiasm and variety of tone!

Active and reflective listening

The skill of active listening is to repeat back to your client what they have said, this should be done frequent enough in order not to forget what has been said, and to confirm what the client is saying. Unless you have practised developing your memory, we usually have the ability to remember around seven things at once, so ensure you jump in at the appropriate moment to reinforce what has been said. Active listening can help to stop your client going off on a tangent; and allow you to confirm what your client has said.
Reflective listening differs from active listening, and it could be described as the process of making an educated guess of what is being said. Reflective listening allows you to focus on what your client is telling you, and to gain an understanding without interrupting; as this can be very distracting for the talker and can often cause loss of concentration; leading to forgetting what they were talking about in the first place. When you are listening, it may help to visualise and picture what is being said, and this can help to understand what is being said. Your role during reflective listening is to analyse and interpret what is being said, so once the talker has finished, take a moment to process the final pieces of information and do not rush to reply, then, when you are ready, reply by giving your understanding of the conversation. Always show empathy and

understanding when listening to your client and commenting back in response, this will help build trust between your client and you.

Building rapport

Building rapport is most important when meeting new clients, it simply means to build a relationship with someone that you have never met, and it's the 'getting to know someone' stage that is vital for making the first impression. There is no particular mode of conversation used for rapport building, but usually relaxed and informal conversation is best; rather than jumping straight into the conversation and run the risk of the client feeling anxious, intimidated or under pressure. So many times I have seen fitness instructors go straight into a session with a client without making any effort to build that initial rapport, even if the session is only for an hour or less and it is unlikely that the instructor will work with the client again, it is still really important to make an effort.

Stages of change

The stage of change model was originally devised by Prochaska and DiClemente (1983) to assist and assess people giving up smoking by identifying and removing or reducing a negative behaviour, however, it has become widely used for other areas of health and well-being; including physical activity. At each stage, a particular behaviour change has to be accomplished in order to move on to the next stage. For personal trainers and the fitness industry it can help to assess where somebody is mentally at in relation to physical activity, and assist in the programming process. Identifying where a client is at is not their role, but rather yours, as it is up to you to question them, and based on their attitude and current exercise habits, make a judgement, and decide at which stage they are at. Below gives you an overview of each stage:

Pre-contemplation

The client has no intention of changing their behavior or becoming physically active at this stage. They have not thought about it at all, they may be aware of change but may have no motivation to change.

Contemplation

At this stage the client has thought about change and may be considering partaking in exercise or being more physically active. They may have been looking into the benefits of exercise and spoken to friends and family who do regularly participate in regular activity.

Preparation

During the preparation stage, the potential exerciser will begin to make plans regarding exercise, for example; they may book a gym induction, buy some new exercise clothing, or even have a consultation with a personal trainer.

Action

This is the point in which an individual makes their first step to changing their behaviour by literally 'taking action' and they have become active on a regular basis. Plenty of motivation is required here in order to keep the client focused and interested. This is the stage in which most people will back out and give up.

Maintenance

The client has remained physically active (behaviour change) for at least six months and they begin to consider this as 'usual behaviour'. Support is required at this stage to ensure that relapse doesn't occur.

Termination

The termination stage indicates that the exerciser has integrated this new behaviour into their lifestyle; and they no longer engage in their old behaviour.

Relapse

Relapse can occur at any stage, and the exerciser may revert back to their old ways, however, it usually occurs during the action and maintenance stage. Your clients may continuously move back and forth through these stages and may find it hard to make exercise a permanent part of their life.

Chapter 4

Fitness assessment and posture analysis

The assessment of somebody's health and fitness is an important part of any programme design; which will also help to manage their fitness programme over a period of time. The American College of Sports Medicine (ACSM) advocate fitness testing for the following reasons:
- Provides you the trainer and the client with a starting point to work from
- Educates the client regarding their fitness
- Enhances motivation towards their exercise regime and progress

There are other reasons why fitness testing is a good idea, for the client, and the trainer; such as, professionalism, helps programme design and a form of screening.

VARTEC

When we are considering carrying out fitness assessments, one thing we need to be aware of is that we can carry out each test exactly the same way every time, to ensure we gain correct, accurate and reliable results. Therefore, we need to consider an acronym known as VARTEC.

VALIDITY – Does the test measure what you want it to? This may sound obvious, but we need to consider the principle of specificity here, and the more specific we can be, the better. So let's assume that our client wants to increase their 10k race time, the best way to test this is to get our client to run 10,000 metres, and ideally on a running track. We could do it on a treadmill if a running track was unavailable, but running on a treadmill is much different to running outside. This is going to be a bench mark if improving time is the goal; run the distance and measure the time taken, simple.

ACCURACY – How accurate is the test that you are doing? Will it give a true result? If we use our 10k example, then yes! We have a 10,000 metre track, and a stopwatch, this is going to be very accurate. However, consider the use of equipment, bio-electrical impedance device, particularly the hand held unit, which passes an electrical current from one hand to another, and based on the speed of the current, an estimation of body fat is measured, less accurate compared to a hand to foot device, this will give a 'more' accurate reading than a handheld unit, as it passes through more of the body. There are far more accurate ways of measuring body fat and these include the use of skin fold callipers and underwater weighing.

RELIABILITY – If the test is repeated, will it be done the same way as before, and whether it is administered by the same person or someone different, we need to ensure the test will be carried out in the same way. Sometimes, depending on the circumstances of the personal trainer, and/or the venue, a different person may have to deliver the test, so the question is; will both parties be able to deliver the test the same? Something like the 10,000 metres is going to be quite straight forward, but consider the use of skin fold callipers and body fat testing, this is quite a skilful test to deliver and it may differ from person to person.

TIME – Some fitness tests are very quick and simple, and on the other hand some are very timely. So my advice for this is that; if you are going to deliver tests that take a long time, ensure that they are totally appropriate for the client and are worth the time spent on them. I do remember when I first started delivering fitness assessments to clients, I would spend a whole hour trying to squeeze in as many tests as possible, and now I know that this resulted in a waste of time on a whole bunch of tests that my client didn't even need. It might even be that there are some tests that measure the same thing and take a lesser amount of time, however, then you may have to refer back to the accuracy of the test, either way, you decide on what you think is best for your client.

EQUIPMENT – Unless you have access to lots of equipment, you may find it a good idea to consider tests that don't need too much equipment, particularly if you are going to be visiting clients in their own home. I would recommend a minimal amount of fitness testing and health assessment equipment, so don't think you'll be ok without any equipment and delivering no tests. There are many tests that you can deliver without the use of equipment, and many of these tests you may also make up yourself, as long as it does what it is supposed to. Some equipment can be quite big and bulky, for example the sit and reach box, used for measuring hamstring and back flexibility, it is a rather large piece of equipment, not really the kind of thing you want to be carrying to your clients house, particularly not if you have other fitness equipment to carry, I have found the use of a step is a great and simple way to measure flexibility as the sit and reach box does.

COST – The main influencing factor on the type of equipment you have is the cost. In most cases the more money you spend on specialised equipment the more accurate the results you are going to get, but specialised fitness testing equipment is very expensive, and with the expense comes size and bulkiness, so unless you have the money and the studio space to store it in, you may find yourself opting for the cheaper options. But let's not assume that if the test equipment is cheap then the test results are not accurate, because there are many tests you could perform and gain very accurate results from, and many you could do with just the use of a stopwatch.

Components of physical fitness

As fitness professionals it is really important to know the different components of physical fitness in which our clients may want to improve. They may not have very clear goals and therefore may also have no idea of which component of fitness they want to achieve, they may know how they want to feel but struggle to identify this in relation to fitness.

Total fitness encompasses a range of components that are outside the realms of this book, and as a personal trainer we focus mainly on physical and nutritional fitness, however, we also need to consider spiritual, mental, social and medical fitness in relation to our client and their goals.

The sub components of physical fitness are as follows; cardiovascular fitness, muscular strength, muscular endurance, flexibility and motor skills. Let's look at these in a little more detail to give you a clearer understanding.

Cardiovascular fitness

This component of fitness is related to the breathlessness you feel whilst participating in planned or unplanned physical activity, for example, if I decide to mow the lawn and do some vigorous gardening, depending on how hard or intense I am working, this would be working my cardiovascular system, or if I decided to go for a run, or a bike ride, this would also work my cardiovascular system.

The cardiovascular system composes of the lungs, the heart and the circulatory system (blood vessels). Cardiovascular fitness is defined as the amount of oxygen you can take in, circulate or transport and utilise. This is known as VO2 max, which stands for maximum volume of oxygen, and it is measured as ml/kg bodyweight/min.

But to help with understanding and to make things easier, let me try and explain things in a different way. We breathe in approximately 21% oxygen with each breath of air that we take, that air is drawn into the lungs, predominantly by the diaphragm, to the air sacks in the lungs called the alveoli, this is where a process called diffusion takes place and oxygen is extracted from the alveoli into the blood vessels; then carried to the heart. It is the hearts responsibility to transport the oxygen rich blood to the rest of the body and particularly the muscles, and at this site the oxygen will be extracted and used to fuel the aerobic energy system, and more importantly keep the muscles working. The breathlessness that you feel when you are working on your cardiovascular fitness is the increase and build-up of carbon dioxide in the blood, a by-product of aerobic training, your body registers this and in response increases breathing rate to help disperse this carbon dioxide. The increase in heart rate is to keep up with the demand of oxygen to the muscle for fuel.

Muscular endurance

For anyone who is active; there will be a repetitious action of muscles contracting and changing length during physical activity, for example, gardening requires continuous and repetitious movements depending on the type of gardening you are doing, but from experience using a flymo lawn mower would work your arms and abdominals over an extended period of time, likewise, if you attend body conditioning classes, you perform many repetitions of different resistance exercises. These are examples of muscular endurance, and the definition for this is; the ability to overcome a sub-maximal resistance over a prolonged period of time, and an example of this could be to perform 20 press ups without stopping.
Depending on the intensity, it is usually during muscular endurance training when you will experience an uncomfortable burning sensation in the muscle, this is known as lactic acid, however it is caused by hydrogen ions, which is a by-product of the anaerobic lactic acid energy system, and after a period of time; and once blood lactate levels reach a certain level, muscle contraction will be inhibited, forcing the exerciser to either reduce the intensity in which they are working at, or stop completely.

In my experience as a personal trainer, I have never had anyone say to me that they want to improve their muscular endurance as one of their goals, that's not to say I have never trained anyone for muscular endurance, cause the fact is that every client I have ever trained has done some kind of muscular endurance, it's just that the majority of people associate weight training and lifting weights with gaining strength and size, and perhaps are not really aware of the term muscular endurance.

Muscular strength

Improving strength is a very common goal expressed by clients, they may state that they just want to be stronger generally, or they may come to you with a very specific strength goal or area of the body that they want to improve and get stronger, either way they want to improve muscular strength. When discussing muscular strength, we often use the term 1RM (repetition maximum), it means the maximum amount of weight you can lift only once, regardless of which area of the body you are testing; for example, if I was to use the leg press machine and only perform one repetition maximum, I would need to select a weight that only allowed me to lift it once, meaning it is too heavy for me to perform a second repetition, this would be a true demonstration of strength in my legs on the leg press. We could however isolate muscles depending on whether we have the appropriate equipment that works individual muscles in isolation, but it would still be specific to that particular machine.

If a client expresses interest in strength as part of their exercise and fitness goals, would it be appropriate to give them 1RM on a selection of machines? Of course not, that would be completely inappropriate, especially for a beginner to exercise, however, sport specific training may require the athlete to perform a 1RM depending on the sport itself, and this is where the principle of specificity comes into play.

Flexibility

The sad and simple fact is that on average, only half the people who exercise stretch effectively at the end of their workout, and the consequence of not stretching as part of your exercise regime can lead to tight, inflexible muscles with a reduced range of movement and a higher risk of flexibility related injuries. So what do we need to do about this then? Well I'm sure you answered correctly, to include flexibility and stretching within our exercise session.

The definition of flexibility is as follows, 'the range of movement around a joint'. Therefore, flexibility only relates to the joints of the body, and usually synovial joints, these joints can be found at the ankle, knee, hip, elbow and knee, often referred to as a 'freely moveable' joint. A synovial joint has the characteristics of; a joint capsule, synovial fluid and articular cartilage at the ends of the two bones that meet to form the joint itself. Flexibility and range of movement can be reduced and inhibited by a number of factors, these include; joint structure, excessive tissue around the joint, tight muscles and injury.

Motor skills

A skill is something you can learn and improve, a toddler will spend months learning to walk, learning the skills of balance and co-ordination, as grown-ups we have developed the skill very well over many years and can do it with perfect technique, it comes naturally and we don't even need to think about it. Driving is also another very good example of learning skills, as you're learning to drive you have a mass of thought and action processes that are taking place, often leaving you soaking with perspiration due to the stress involved. If you have been driving for a few years you may find yourself somewhere without remembering the journey, your driving has become automatic.

It has been discovered that visualising a movement pattern in your mind will actually help you to improve that movement for real. By doing this, it is believed that the neuromuscular pathways used to perform the movement are stimulated; this allows you to become skilled at the movement as new nerve connections are made.

When discussing motor skills, we are referring to the motor neurons or nerves of the nervous system. It is the job of the nervous system, even more importantly, motor units, to send electrical and chemical messages to the working muscle. These signals are sent via the central nervous system in response to a variety of external and internal stimuli.
We possess a number of motor skills and for different activities and different sports we participate in, we require these motor skills in differing amounts. Let's identify the motor skills to obtain a better understanding.

Balance – maintaining position whilst keeping centre of gravity

Agility – changing direction with speed

Co-ordination – moving parts of the body in a particular controlled order

Reaction time – speed of response to an audible, visual or physical stimulus

Speed – the speed in which a single or continuous movement can be executed

Power - Power is often listed as a motor skill, however, power is a combination of speed and strength and is equated as velocity x force. If person A can push a car 20 meters in 30 seconds and person B can push the same distance in 20 seconds, person B is considered having more power. Power output is the greatest when speed and resistance are set to the highest level, see the following diagram.

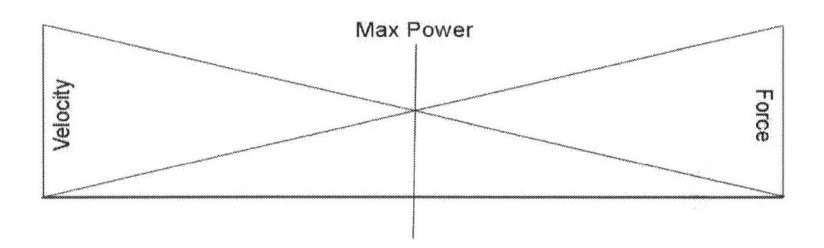

Fitness testing

It is really important to deliver fitness tests that are specific to the clients' goals; for example, it would be pointless to give your client tests for cardiovascular fitness if their only goal was to increase muscular strength. So the answer to the question that I get asked frequently when lecturing on this topic is, 'which fitness tests should I give my client?' the answer is simple, the tests that directly relate to the clients goals.

For this section we are going to look at a number of fitness tests that we can deliver to our clients, and also identify the advantages and disadvantages of each. With a better understanding, this will help you to choose appropriate tests to give your clients, enabling you to effectively monitor and assess your client's progress.

Cardiovascular

Aerobic or cardiovascular fitness is measured as VO2 max, and this simply refers to the amount of oxygen an individual can take in, transport and utilise.

There are number of well known tests to assess cardiovascular fitness, one of the most common is the bleep test, the bleep test is a progressive maximum test which can last up to 20 minutes depending on the fitness of the individual. The idea of the bleep test is to run between two markers set at 20 metres apart, following a set pattern of bleeps that speed up after every minute. The bleep test starts off quite slow, this allows you to gradually warm up, you must end the test when you are no longer able to keep up with the set rhythm and record the level and how many shuttles you have completed, so your result may look something like 12.6 (level 12, shuttle 6). The results from this test can be compared to a norm chart and can also be used to estimate your VO2 max.

The Cooper test is also a very popular fitness test, it is a twelve minute run at your fastest sustainable speed, you will obviously need a treadmill or a running track to measure the distance and a stopwatch to keep track of time, similar to the bleep test, you can check your score with a norm chart and also estimate your VO2 max.

If your client is unable to run, the Rockport test is ideal; this test requires a treadmill and a heart rate monitor. The idea of the Rockport test is to walk at your fastest sustainable speed for the distance of one mile, or 1.61km, whichever your treadmill displays. You must measure the time taken and record the heart rate just before you reach your distance. With this information recorded and your clients' weight and age, you will then be able to do the appropriate calculation for determining estimated VO2 max.

The YMCA step test is a great fitness test if you do not have access to a gym or treadmill, all you require is a 12 inch step, a metronome and a stop watch. The idea of this test is to step up and down for three minutes to the sound of the metronome set at 96bpm. After three minutes, recovery heart rate has to be recorded for one minute and compared to the norm chart. This test does not assess VO2 max, it measures recovery rate, and the quicker your heart rate comes down after exercise, the fitter you are (for most people), so by counting the amount of heart beats in a minute after exercise you are able to monitor fitness level.

Muscular strength and endurance

Maximal strength or 1RM testing is not generally recommended for beginners as their skeleton and skeletal muscles may not be accustomed to the type of stress you can expect from this degree of resistance. So for strength testing beginners, we tend to choose a repetition range between 6 and 8, and this gives us a much safer and functional result.
For the more experience exerciser, it would be more appropriate to test maximal strength, but only if the client expressed their desire to do so, otherwise I would still stick with the 6-8. When testing 1RM's ensure your client is appropriately warm and a few light sets of the exercise you are using have been executed, this will help to warm up the muscle being tested and the joint associated with the exercise to help prevent injury.
Assessing muscular endurance is much easier than assessing strength, and is also much safer as it requires many more reps over a longer period with a lighter weight. There are a couple of different ways in which to do this, the weight you can lift over a set number of repetitions, for example; what is the maximum weight you can lift for 20-25 repetitions. Or you could test the number of repetitions completed at a set weight over a period of time, say one minute.

Flexibility and range of movement

Flexibility assessment is an excellent way of identifying someone's range of movement around a joint and can also assist in posture analysis and assist in the correction process. Tight and shortened muscles can create tension and pain, and also affect posture, so delivering a flexibility assessment can instantly help to identify these issues. The most common flexibility test is the sit and reach test, designed to assess the flexibility of your upper and lower back, and also hamstrings. You are required to sit on the floor with straight legs and your bare feet flat against the step, and without bending your knees you lean forward from the hips and reach as far forward as you can with control, the distance is measured over three attempts and the best result is recorded. The result is measured in centremetres beyond foot level. The result must be compared to the norm chart, but can also be used as a bench mark if doing it for the first time.

Testing flexibility and range of movement for other areas, the use of a goniometer is a good idea in order to measure the exact angle of the relative joint. If this equipment is unavailable, then observation of angle and position is still an effective way of measuring range of movement. The most important thing to consider when assessing range of movement is the ability for your client to maintain good posture and spinal alignment, if this is not maintained throughout, then the measurements and results become inaccurate. Flexibility around joints can also be compared to each other; i.e. left arm and right arm.

Relative strength

When we talk about being strong, we tend to relate it to the amount of weight that is lifted, and as the definition states, strength is the ability to overcome or lift a maximal weight for one repetition, known as 1RM. Having a large muscle mass and being able to lift a considerable amount of weight clearly demonstrates a high degree of strength, however, if we compare the amount of weight lifted to the weight of the individual, then the degree of strength may not actually be as high as we thought, and this is the theory behind relative strength; the amount of weight lifted in relation to body weight.
If person A weighs 120kg and their 1RM on the bench press is 200kg, and person B weighs 80kg and their 1RM on the bench press is 150kg, then person B is considered stronger in relative strength. An example of this is also seen in the gym when you see a muscle bound weight lifter using plenty of weight on a lat pull down machine, but may struggle and find it difficult to lift their own body weight during chin ups.

Having a higher strength to weight ratio is much more functional for day to day living, and can make daily activities and tasks much easier, so functional or relative strength is what we should be focusing on unless we have a specific sporting goal or just want to be bigger generally.
Being bigger doesn't necessarily mean getting stronger; the body adapts differently to size and strength training. Being stronger is

associated with an efficient neuromuscular nervous system, and the ability to recruit a maximum number of motor units for any given task. Having larger (cross section) muscle fibres will help to gain further strength, and for some people, strength to weight ratio can be maintained, however, for others gaining hypertrophy (muscle size) is much easier, and this is where a balance of strength and weight control should be considered.

What else can we assess?

The above are related to physical fitness, and it is considered you are in good shape if you possess a good level of each component of physical fitness. We also need to consider other elements of fitness which people may possess that are not actually related to exercise; as mentioned earlier, these are nutritional, social, medical, mental and spiritual fitness, all of these plus physical fitness make up 'total fitness' taking these other factors into consideration are really important when assessing somebody's physical fitness.

Health assessment

As well as physical fitness, it is also very important to assess someone's general health, and the following will identify what you can assess and what it means.

Body Mass Index (BMI)

Body Mass Index (BMI) is a very useful way of determining whether someone is overweight by comparing their weight to height, and can be calculated by using the following formula and checking it against the norm chart below. BMI = weight (kilos) divided by height squared (metres).

	BMI
Underweight	<18.5
Normal	18.6-24.9

Overweight	25-29.9
Obese	30>

(ACSM 2006)

What BMI cannot do is distinguish the difference between lean mass (muscle, bone and organs) and body fat; therefore, if you were to use it on someone who has a visually large amount of muscle mass and little body fat, it will no doubt indicate that this particular individual is either overweight or even obese. With this in mind it is very important to take other factors into consideration when using BMI and not to use it as a means of measuring body fat or body composition.

Anthropometric measurements

Anthropometry roughly translates as 'man' and 'measure', and it refers to the measurements of the human body for the understanding of human physical variation.
In the field of ergonomics, anthropometry is used to optimise the design and use of equipment and environments.

Taking girth measurements are an excellent way of identifying changes in body composition. This type of assessment can be very motivating for clients who either want to lose or increase size; the procedure is very easy, reproducible, reliable and cheap, and only a tape measure is needed. Care must be taken to ensure the tape is level and even around the area being measured, the exact same spot is used to measure, and also an accurate reading is taken.

The use of a tape measure can help you to see a clearer picture regarding someone's health. Simply by taking waist and hip circumferences we can collect more accurate information. There is very clear evidence to show that high body fat levels (particularly around the abdomen) are closely related to Coronary Heart Disease (CHD), as well as some cancers, diabetes and stroke. A simple waist measurement can be taken on its own and compared to the norm chart below, however, because people come in all different shapes and sizes, it is inaccurate to assume that this chart can be used for everyone. However, the primary healthcare system have adopted the use of waist measurement on its own as an indicator of poor health, as there is an established correlation between the two.

Risk Category	Females	Males
Very low	<70	<80
Low	70-89	80-99
High	90-109	100-120
Very high	>110	>120

(ACSM 2006)

Waist to hip ratio

This particular anthropometric measurement is a very reliable indicator of high fat levels and therefore people who are at high risk of developing CHD. By comparing the waist and hip measurements, we can calculate whether someone is carrying excess body fat around their midriff, as waist measurement should be smaller than hip measurement. The relationship between excessive body fat around the abdomen and CHD is very evident, making this test very appropriate for most people. Divide the waist by the hip measurement and then check the recommendation below to find out if you are at a recommended and safe level. You are classified at high risk if your waist to hip ratio exceeds the following:

Waist
Hips

Males 0.94
Females 0.82

Waist and hip measurement alone can also be used as a very effective measurement to monitor progress in body fat loss. If used in conjunction with body composition, it can give a much clearer and definitive result.

Blood pressure

In my opinion, taking someone's blood pressure before any physical activity takes place is the most important part of health assessment. There is a very large number of people who are being let into a gym (and exercise classes) without having their blood pressure taken, and those who do have it done may be pre-hypertensive (above normal) or even worse, have hypertension (high blood pressure).

Blood pressure is the measurement of force exerted on the artery walls during the two phases of the heart cycle, these are systole and diastole, when the heart beats and relaxes respectively. Blood pressure is measured by cutting off circulation, usually at the brachial artery in the upper arm by the use of a cuff that is pumped with air to exert high pressure around your arm. The pressure is gradually released until blood can pass through at a very slightly higher pressure than that of the cuff; this is recorded as systolic pressure. As the pressure is further reduced, the point in which there is no resistance to the cuff is the diastolic pressure, and this measurement is also recorded. The pressure is measured in mmHg (millimetres of mercury) by a sphygmomanometer and stethoscope.
Blood pressure can be measured manually as above, and can also be taken electronically by an automatic unit. The latter is much easier and more user friendly than taking it manually. Taking blood pressure manually requires much experience before an accurate measurement can be assumed.
Automatic blood pressure monitors are widely available these days, with more and more people buying them for their own use.

BP classification	Systole BP (mmHg)	Diastole BP (mmHg)
Normal	<120	And <80
Pre-hypertension	120-139	Or 80-89
Stage1 hypertension	140-159	Or 90-99
Stage2 hypertension	>160	Or >100

Norms for blood pressure (ACSM 2006)

When taking your clients blood pressure, ensure you follow the correct protocol in order to gain accurate readings. Blood pressure is influenced by many factors; including stress, caffeine, nicotine, lack of sleep and other stimulants. Taking someone's blood pressure two or three times is advisable as anxiety will increase it temporarily, this is known as the white coat syndrome and you may be familiar with this from when you last visited the dentist or the doctors. It's an automatic response from the sympathetic nervous system that prepares us for stressful situations, not always very useful though, especially when someone tells you not to worry!

Some people have low blood pressure (below normal), this doesn't pose any health risks; however, your client may suffer from dizziness when moving from position to position, particularly from the floor and off a CV machine. Ensure you discuss this with your client if they haven't exercised before. The main concern you both have is the risk of your client injuring themselves due to passing out.

If your blood pressure is 140-159 and/or 90-99 you are considered to be stage 1 hypertensive, your doctor will recommend lifestyle changes and probably prescribe a diuretic medication to lower the fluid and sodium in the blood.

If your blood pressure is 160 or above and/or 100 or above you are considered to be stage 2 hypertensive, at this stage, people must make lifestyle changes and take 2 types of medication, a diuretic and an antihypertensive drug, a third medication may need to be prescribed if necessary.

Regular cardiovascular exercise can help normalise blood pressure for certain individuals, this means either bringing it down slightly (approximately 10mmHg) or increasing it slightly if it is low. Avoid telling people that exercise brings blood pressure down, because if their blood pressure is already low, they may not like the prospect of lowering it even more and therefore not be excited by the thought of exercise.

A final thought here, when taking blood pressure and feeding back the result to your client; remember we cannot diagnose high blood pressure, we can only inform someone that they have elevated blood pressure and they should get it checked out by their GP.

Heart rate

Resting heart rate is a general way of identifying an individual's cardiovascular fitness. As your cardiovascular fitness improves, and your heart becomes stronger and able to pump more blood per beat, this is known as stroke volume. If your heart can pump more blood per beat, it has to beat less frequently (less bpm) in order to pump the same amount of blood per minute, this is called cardiac output.
Resting heart rate is generally between 60 and 80bpm, and the average is 72bpm.
Measuring heart rate can give you an idea of as to how their health is improving over a period of weeks.
Some elite athletes have resting heart rates as low as 30, we wouldn't expect our clients to get as low as that, but we can certainly use it to monitor the effectiveness of their training.

Body composition

Body composition is a popular assessment amongst exercisers and people interested in weight management. When discussing body composition, we are actually referring to two different aspects of body composition, these are body fat and lean tissue. If someone weighs 70kgs and they have 20 percent body fat, the other 80 percent is considered lean tissue. Knowing the above information means you can calculate the weight of each. 20 percent of 70 is 14 (14kgs fat) and 80 percent of 70 is 56 (56kgs lean tissue).

There are several ways in which to measure body fat and body composition, including underwater weighing and DEXA Scanner which stands for dual energy x-ray absorptiometry. These are expensive and not easily accessed methods, but they are some of the most accurate.
Methods used within a fitness environment include skin-fold callipers and bioelectrical impedance devices. It is very common for most gyms to have this equipment and use it on a regular basis as part of clients programming and fitness assessment.
The use of skin fold callipers is the more accurate of the two; but does take a while to perform; it also takes experience to ensure the

most accurate results. It is advisable that the same person carries out this test on an individual client, as a different trainer may do it very slightly different.

The principle of using this technique is that by taking measurements of subcutaneous fat from various areas of the body are proportionate to the total amount of body fat. The measurements of skin fold are added together and are used to estimate total body fat.

It is not always appropriate to use this form of body composition testing; for example, it would not give an accurate reading for an obese client, it may also be very invasive for some people who didn't want to expose any part of their body to you. So do ensure you fully explain the protocol for this test with your client before you go jumping in pinching their skin and fat!

As well as giving an accurate estimation of body fat percentage, the use of skin fold measurements can also act as a bench mark. Because you have to accurately mark the site in which you are measuring, we can simply use this site and reading to compare to skin fold readings that are done in 6-8 weeks time when we re-measure. This will give us a very accurate reading of whether we have shed any body fat and to what extent.

A much easier way to assess body composition is the use of a bioelectrical impedance device. The principle behind this form of assessment is that a low electrical current is passed through the body, and judging by the speed and resistance to the current, an approximate body fat percentage is calculated.

The three most common devices are Bodystat®, Tanita® and Omron®.

Bodystat® uses a set of electrodes attached to the hand and wrist and another set attached to the foot and ankle of the same side of the body. The client must lie in a horizontal position as the current runs through the body. This appears to be the most accurate of the three as it travels furthest and through the upper 'and' lower body.

Tanita® is a popular device and found in many people's bathrooms, they look just like a regular set of scales, but with electrodes in the form of metal plates on either side. You stand on the device with bare feet as the current is passed from one foot through the lower body to the other foot. Here the current only passes through the lower body, avoiding the upper body. This method is fine as long as you haven't got a disproportionate amount of body fat in the upper body compared to the lower body.

Omron® is the most popular with gyms as it doesn't require you to lie down, nor does it require you to take off any clothing, it is also the cheapest option. This device is handheld, and similar to the Tanita® device, but has electrodes on the hand grips. You hold the device out in front of you as the current passes from one hand, through the upper body and to the other hand. Here the current only passes through the upper body, avoiding the lower body, therefore the same rules apply as the above device.

Pre-assessment guidelines

Before you begin any health and fitness testing, there are a number of things to consider and to make your client aware of, ensuring that the tests are as accurate as possible and the whole procedure runs smoothly.

Trainer considerations:
- Have your testing area room ready and arranged appropriately
- Try and conduct each health and fitness assessment at the same time of day
- Follow the correct protocol for each test
- Ensure all your equipment is clean and in good working order
- Have all norm charts and recording paperwork available
- Begin with health assessment, i.e. blood pressure and body composition
- Cardiovascular fitness, muscular strength and endurance should be performed last

Client considerations:
- Avoid any stimulants within at least 3 hours of testing
- Wear appropriate clothing, loose and comfortable
- Aim to get 6-8 hours sleep the night before
- Avoid strenuous exercise or stress before the test

- Ensure adequate energy by eating 3 hours before
- Stay hydrated by drinking plenty of water 24 hours before

Postural analysis

Another area of our clients' health and fitness we can assess is posture. This is a really simple but yet professional service to offer your clients. Generally we are looking for good joint alignment throughout the body from a front and side view. One term we do use to describe posture and specifically to the spine and vertebrae is neutral spine.

The spine has a number of natural curves throughout its length in the sagittal plane, meaning you can clearly see from a side. One of the main reasons for this curvature is to absorb shock from forces through the lower body reaching the cranium. Everybody has these curves, however, not everyone's spinal curves are going to be the same, our job when assessing posture is to check, record and monitor any changes or major issues. Although we have identified that people have varying degrees of curvature of the spine, we also need to be aware that there are conditions of over-curvature of the spine. For example; the area of the spine which is attached to the ribs is the thoracic vertebrae, and is convex from a posterior context, this means if you look at somebody's area of back where the ribs are, their back will 'stick out' slightly, and the hunchback of Notre Dame is a perfect example of this. When an over-curvature occurs of the thoracic spine, it tends to take the spine out of neutral alignment, and this condition is called kyphosis. The lower spine consists of the five lumbar vertebrae, this also has a natural curve in it; this is convex from an anterior aspect, i.e. from the front. The lumbar curve can be seen and often quite prominent when the backside is pushed out. An over-curvature of the lumbar spine is called lordosis; this is very common during pregnancy due to the large amount of weight carried to the front of the lower spine. Some people can naturally have an exaggerated lumbar curve and is also common amongst Afro-Caribbean communities.

When observing posture from the side, the use of a plumb line is very useful, when lined up with the ankle, it should then line up with the knee, hip joint, shoulder joint and ear. Most people will have some degree of imbalance, so it's then our job to identify what needs to be prescribed in order to rectify the issue. An imbalance will include tight shortened muscles and weak lengthened muscles; however, a lengthened muscle does not necessarily mean it is weak.

As well as observing our client from side, we should consider observing them from the front and back too. When we observe and assess from the front, we are looking for any areas of the body which are not level, for example, the neck, shoulders or hips, and if this is the case, there is likely to be a degree of scoliosis occurring (S type lateral curvature). Other areas that should be observed and checked for symmetry are; pectoral lines, distal ends of the quads, gluteal lines, calf line and scapula, you should also check foot alignment and any pronation or supination.

Spinal conditions

The spine or vertebral column is a combination of 33 vertebrae, mostly separated by cartilaginous vertebral discs, and they run from the base of the skull to the tail bone (coccyx). The spinal column holds and protects the spinal cord (part of the central nervous system). The spinal column has a number of curves in it, this is to act as a shock absorber for the skull and brain, each person's curvature of the spine is different, but essentially all act for the same purpose. Neutral spine is a term used to describe everybody's individual but optimum and natural curvature of the spine. Through daily living and incorrect posture; we can end up abusing these natural curves and unfortunately they change and alter, leading us into over-curvature of different areas of the spine, and leaving us with an imbalance of muscles and often discomfort and pain.

Lordosis

Lordosis occurs in the lower (lumbar) spine between the ribs and the pelvis. From an anterior view, this curve of the lumbar spine is convex (the apex of the curve protrudes forward). Lordosis can be described as an over-curvature of the lumbar spine; which can be caused during pregnancy, excessive weight around the abdomen and bad posture, but is also common amongst certain ethnic groups and can exaggerate the size of the backside.

One of the major issues associated with lordosis is a herniated vertebral disc, this is due to uneven pressure on each vertebrae, and causes the cartilaginous disc to push onto the nerves, especially the largest nerve in the body; the sciatic nerve that runs down each leg, causing leg pain, known as sciatica.

Kyphosis

Kyphosis occurs in the mid section of the spine, known as the thoracic spine, and each vertebrae in this section is attached to a rib. Over-curvature of the thoracic spine is characterised by a hunchback type posture and is very common in growing teenagers and tall people, but can also be caused by poor posture, particularly sitting hunched over a desk. The elderly are usually prone to this spinal condition, this is due to the degeneration of the vertebrae and also constantly looking down at the floor to prevent a fall.

Strengthening the thoracic erector spinae (spinal column extensor muscle) and trapezius muscle of the upper back would be recommended to help improve and prevent this condition; however, caution and doctor consent should be gained before treating teenagers and the elderly. The vertebrae in teenagers are not fully formed anteriorly causing a forward lean, and in the elderly the bones of the vertebrae may be damaged, worn away and possibly fused.

Scoliosis

Scoliosis is best described as an abnormal s-shaped lateral curve of the spine and can be either genetic or caused through an imbalance of muscle tone and length. It was once thought to be a childhood disease, but is becoming increasingly common in older adults. Visual signs of scoliosis can be a prominent side of the hip, one shoulder higher or lower than the other, and also leaning to one side.

In adults, the first line of treatment for scoliosis may be pain killers to relieve the painful symptoms. Research into exercise for the treatment of scoliosis has not proven to aid or hinder the symptoms of this condition, but does contribute to a healthy lifestyle and is therefore recommended.

Screening and Informed Consent

One of the most important aspects of personal training is to provide safe, effective and knowledgeable training sessions, always putting your client first, delivering excellent customer care, and remaining professional. Without these, I have no doubt that you are destined to fail as a personal trainer, sorry! Focusing for now on the safe and effective; we must discuss the screening process that has to take place with you and your client. To explain the meaning of screening in just a few words, I would have to say, it is the process of ensuring your client is ready to exercise. Just for a moment, imagine meeting a client for the first time you know nothing about, you ask no questions and they tell you nothing about themselves, and without wasting any time, you proceed to take them through an exercise regime you put together before the session began and even meeting this client. Now there are two issues here, the first issue is that you have no idea of their goals or what they want to achieve, we won't discuss this now as it is covered in another chapter, but issue two, is that we have no idea where they have come from, any injuries they may have, medical conditions, capabilities, concerns and any other issues we did not allow them to express. So hopefully now you see the purpose of screening, it is the most important thing you do before you start anyone on a programme of physical activity.

The screening process should take place prior to, and during exercise, and a pre-activity readiness questionnaire (PARQ) should be completed by the client before exercise commences. A PARQ usually consists of approximately 7 or 8 very specific questions relating to the clients health status, for example; heart problems, bone or joint issues etc. This type of screening doesn't always give you the whole picture of someone's health and fitness; so further verbal screening is required, either at the time of the PARQ being completed, or by the trainer before exercise begins, this really depends on the set up of the gym and or whether you are the first point of contact to the client.

Verbal screening is very quick and simple to do, it just requires you to ask your client a few key questions, such as; "how are you feeling today?", "do you have any injuries I need to know about that might affect your participation in exercise?", "has anything changed since you completed your PARQ?" This type of questioning should ideally be done for each individual client before the start of every exercise session, just to ensure they are fit to exercise. Verbal screening is a very informal way of ensuring your client is ok to exercise, so be certain the questions you ask give you a clear picture of that.

Remember, a written PARQ is only valid for that moment it is completed. In theory; once it has been completed it then becomes invalid! So, how often should a PARQ be completed? Ideally, every session, but as you can imagine this is not practical, and it is also a waste of paper. I would recommend every six months if you continue to see your client on a regular basis, and after a period of not seeing your client or them not exercising is definitely a wise idea. The fact that you screened your client before exercise may not be a 'get out of jail card' if unfortunately things do go wrong, but it will show you had and demonstrated a duty of care towards your client, and may save you from being declared negligent, in the unlikely event that something did go wrong.

Chapter 5

Medical conditions

The following section has been put together to give you an idea of some of the conditions people may have and you need to be aware of, especially if these people are to become personal training clients. If you aim to work with people who have more serious conditions, then you must obtain an appropriate qualification, this will give you greater knowledge and will also ensure that your insurance will cover you should anything happen while training these particular client groups.

Diabetes Mellitus

Diabetes is the inability of the pancreas to produce and secrete insulin into the blood, causing blood sugar levels to rise dangerously. This is very serious lifelong condition that affects 2.9 million people in the UK, and it is thought that nearly a million people have undiagnosed diabetes. When blood glucose levels are high, and insulin isn't released, or the cells in the body do not respond to the insulin (insulin resistance), high levels of glucose in the blood can cause major damage to the organs of the body, blood vessels and nerves.

There are two types of diabetes, and type 2 is the most common form, that makes up for about 90% of people diagnosed. With type 2 diabetes, the pancreas does not produce enough insulin to adequately draw glucose out of the blood and into the cells of the body, this is called insulin resistance. Type 2 diabetes; more commonly affects people over the age of forty, but more and more people are being diagnosed at a much younger age. Diabetes cannot be cured and is a progressive disease, so therefore if you are diagnosed, it is likely that your condition could become worse.

Once diagnosed, you will be advised to make nutritional changes to help stabilise blood sugar levels and may also be given medication; if your condition does worsen, you may be prescribed insulin.

Type 1 diabetes, or insulin dependent diabetes, is less common and usually develops during teenage years, the pancreas does not produce any insulin and therefore you will have to inject it for the rest of your life. You will need to keep a check on your blood glucose levels, eat a healthy diet and take regular exercise.
This form of diabetes is an auto-immune condition; where the immune system (responsible for fighting disease) attacks the cells of the pancreas as they mistake them as harmful.

There are various symptoms of diabetes, and the following are the most common:
- Feeling tired throughout the day
- Frequently urinating, especially at night
- Feeling very thirsty

Coronary heart disease (CHD)

Coronary heart disease or CHD is the UK's biggest killer, and is responsible for approximately 82,000 deaths per year. The main symptoms of CHD are angina, heart attack and heart failure, although many people may be diagnosed with CHD before any symptoms arise. The build up of fatty deposits in the arteries are responsible for the cause of this disease, this condition is called atherosclerosis, and the fatty deposits are called atheroma. This build up in the arteries reduces the space available for the blood to pass through, therefore increasing blood pressure, and when blood pressure increases the risk of part of the fatty deposit breaking away rises, and if this happens, depending on where it goes, could cause a heart attack or stroke.

Obesity

Obesity is defined as having an excessive amount of body fat in relation to body weight, and although BMI cannot distinguish the difference between lean muscle tissue (LMT) and body fat, a BMI of 30+ is defined as obese. There are many terms to describe obesity and regional fat distribution, the most common types are known as android and gynoid obesity. Localisation of body fat around the upper body is known as android obesity, characterised by the apple shape, and this is common amongst males; and then there is gynoid obesity, which is characterised by the pear shape and most common amongst females, however, some females can have android obesity and some males can have gynoid obesity.

Obesity is a rapidly rising issue in the west, as more and more people are being diagnosed, and in certain countries a massive fifty percent of the population are obese. The main cause to this rising problem is the lack of exercise and activity people undertake, balanced with the amount and type of food they consume. With food becoming more and more readily available and convenient, unfortunately the quality becomes compromised, and the main culprits responsible for this are sugar, salt and fat. These 'added' ingredients serve two purposes; to prolong the shelf life and preserve the food, and also to make it taste nice. Studies have shown a food that has a high and equal amount of fat and sugar gives the most satisfying taste which physiologically encourages us to eat more and not feel full.
Weight loss is a very simple equation, if the calories consumed are less than calories expended, as little as a five hundred calorie deficit per day can lead to a 1lb of weight loss per week.
Obesity is closely linked to CHD, as studies have indicated that high levels of body fat (in relation to body weight) around the abdomen and internal organs (visceral fat) increase the risk of heart attack and stroke. High levels of body fat will increase cholesterol levels, and that will lead to atherosclerosis; a build up of fatty tissue that settles on the inside of the arteries.

Arthritis

Arthritis is a common condition that affects the joints, and it causes pain and inflammation. Around ten million people in the UK alone suffer from arthritis, and unfortunately it is an incurable disease. It usually occurs around the age of fifty, however, it can affect any age group and children are also at risk of developing it. Arthritis can also be caused by injury or another condition of the joint. There are two main types of arthritis; these are osteoarthritis and rheumatoid arthritis. With osteoarthritis, the cartilage (connective tissue that protects, cushions and allows ends of bone to move against each other smoothly) at either end of the bones wears away or becomes damaged, and the consequence is bone rubbing against bone, causing major pain and stiffness around the joint. With rheumatoid arthritis, the immune system attacks the joint; this can break down the bone and cartilage, causing pain, swelling and a reduction in range of movement.

Any treatment for arthritis will not cure the condition but will only slow down the degenerative process. Non-steroidal anti-inflammatory drugs (NSAID's) and corticosteroids are often prescribed, and in more severe cases surgery may be necessary, exercise is also recommended to help deal with the pain and symptoms.

Stress

There is no doubt that at some point in everybody's life, we will be faced with stress, and as we become a much busier nation, stress will always be evident in our lives. The truth is, is that we actually need stress in order to survive, it is what keeps us motivated, striving forward and accomplishing tasks, however, too much stress is not good for us, and over an extended period of time, this can suppress the immune system, and excess stress can lead to further illness; including digestive issues, depression, anxiety, insomnia, hypertension and coronary heart disease (CHD) to name a few.

Stress comes in two forms, physiological and psychological; physical exercises such as running, weight lifting and high intensity aerobic activities are perfect examples of physiological stress that we voluntarily place upon ourselves in order to improve our fitness, whereas psychological stressors include events such as, overworked, bereavement, moving house and family illness.

The body cannot tell the difference between these two types of stress, but what it does do is respond in a way that may not be appropriate for the situation, and this is known as the fight or flight response, which is a built in mechanism of the autonomic nervous system, and it prepares us to deal with threatening situations. It does this by increasing heart rate, breathing rate and energy production. The adrenal glands secrete a number of hormones into the blood to assist in the process of fat utilisation, protein catabolism and carbohydrate conservation.

Hans Selye (1956), a pioneering endocrinologist from Hungary, hypothesised the General Adaptation Syndrome (GAS) theory of stress, and gave a scientific explanation to stress. His model identified three stages of bodily response, these are:

- Stage 1: Alarm

The first stage of stress is when the body prepares itself and initiates the 'fight or flight' response to deal with the stressful situation.

- Stage 2: Resistance

This stage is sometimes referred to as the adaptation phase as internal changes begin to take place, and at this stage we either overcome the stressor or the stress continues and we move to the next stage.

- Stage 3: Exhaustion

At this stage, the stress has been present for an extended period of time, and the body's immune system and ability to resist these stressors has almost diminished, therefore leading to further disease or medical conditions, which could be potentially fatal.

It is worth noting that Hans Selye did not identify stress as being a negative phenomenon related to fear and anxiety, but frequently pointed out that it was a positive one related to joy and pleasure as well.

Anaemia

There are many forms of anaemia but iron deficient anaemia is the most common, which causes shortness of breath, fatigue, tiredness and a pale complexion. The condition is caused by a lack of iron (essential for red blood cell production), this leads to a reduction of red blood cells which store and carry oxygen around the body. For most people with anaemia, taking an iron supplement to boost their levels is the answer which causes no long term problems, although you will need to be monitored, usually on a monthly basis to ensure the condition hasn't worsened and while the underlying cause is identified.

Untreated anaemia can cause illness and infection as it affects the immune system. Extreme cases of anaemia can cause complications which affect the heart and lungs such as higher resting and exercising heart rates and a reduced ability of the heart to pump blood around the body.

A balanced diet will ensure a sufficient amount of iron is consumed, and the following foods are known to have good levels of iron in them:

Dried fruit

Eggs

Nuts and seeds

Cereals fortified with iron

Meat and fish

Pulses

Brown rice

Asthma

Asthma is characterised by the coughing and wheezing of the sufferer, and is caused by the narrowing of the air tubes within the lungs, called the bronchioles. Asthma is a chronic condition that cannot be cured, but can be controlled and managed. Most people with this condition have what is called; atopic asthma, this means they have an allergic reaction to external triggers; such as exercise, dust, animal fur, pollen and cigarette smoke. This reaction causes the airways to swell and constrict the passage of air within it, resulting in a wheezing sound and difficulty breathing. Mucus is also produced from the lining of the airway which makes breathing even harder and causes coughing. For some people, the on-set of asthma is unpredictable and may be triggered by stress or anxiety. Preventative treatment can be used to reverse the effect; however, if the symptoms are severe enough, hospital treatment may be necessary. Treatment and prevention includes medication, lifestyle changes and identifying and avoiding certain triggers.

Asthma is common in young people, but can develop at any age, and according to Asthma UK, 5.4 million people are receiving treatment for asthma; that's 1 in every 12 adults and 1 in every 11 children.

Chapter 6

Fitness principles

Principles of exercise

As a fitness instructor and personal trainer it is important that you are familiar with principles of exercise, these are rules that apply specifically to fitness and must be considered when prescribing and delivering exercise.

Overload

One of the most important principles of exercise is overload, because without overload we would not be able to improve our fitness. We are only able to improve our fitness by stressing the muscular and cardiovascular systems beyond a point in which we are used to. It is not during the exercise we get fitter, it is during the rest we have between exercise sessions and while we are sleeping that we get fitter; as your body works hard to adapt to the stresses placed upon it, ensuring it doesn't have to go through it again, and making it feel a fractional easier next time. The definition of overload is to do more than we are accustomed to, and without doing what we are accustomed to from time to time our bodies would not be able to adapt to this additional stress, and therefore get fitter.

Overtraining

Unlike overload, overtraining is undesirable and something you should stay away from. In fitness terms it means not enough rest during training sessions. As we know already, improvements in fitness and adaptations made by the body happen during rest and sleep. Without this rest we do not allow our body to recover, and eventually something has to give. The main side effect of overtraining is a suppressed immune system; in this state our body's struggle to fight infection, and consequently we can become ill, usually an obvious sign is frequent colds or the inability to fight them off. There are many other characteristics of overtraining; some of these are, lack of motivation, fatigue and tiredness, prone to exercise related injury, plateau in fitness level, irritability and insomnia. It is all too easy to become obsessed with training, when every session counts and no opportunity should be lost, and consequently losing sight of overtraining.

Reversibility

The principle of reversibility states that we cannot store fitness, and fitness is a physiological state that cannot be maintained or improved unless the training stimulus continues. Therefore, if we cease training, our fitness will diminish and progressively be lost. What we must understand is that our body adapts to the stress we place upon it, and if the stress does not exist, then our body will get used to dealing with no stress, and then when the body is expected to work harder due to a stressful situation, for example, run for the bus or lift a heavy object, it struggles!

Plateau

A plateau in your training can be seen as a positive or negative thing, and it simply means your workout is remaining the same with an absence of progression. So for someone who is aiming to progress and improve their fitness level, reaching a plateau is a negative thing and obviously something that needs to be avoided. For someone who doesn't have a goal to reach and are happy with their current fitness with no desire to progress it, then it is a positive thing, they simply want to maintain their level of fitness, so continuing to do the same thing will achieve this.

Kinetic chain exercise

Kinetic chain is referred to as the relationship between the nerves, muscles and bones in order to produce a movement or perform an exercise, these areas of the body work together (as a kinetic chain) to bring about the movement and although we may be guilty of just focusing on the prime mover or muscle involved during an exercise, we should also be focusing on how other areas and muscles of the body are moving and helping us to achieve the movement. The kinetic chain is divided into two categories, these are open kinetic chain and closed kinetic chain, and these terms are used to describe or classify an exercise.

Physiotherapists use this method to determine the most effective type of exercise to prescribe to patients during rehabilitation, and also sports coaches in helping to mimic and improve particular sporting actions through training.

Open kinetic chain exercises would be described as an exercise where your arms or legs are in space and free to move as the rest of your body remains still. Many open kinetic chain exercises are of an isolation (single joint) nature; however, this is not always the case, and some publications you read may suggest that open kinetic chain exercises come with a higher risk of injury due to the increase of weight added at the distal end of the limb, therefore increasing resistance considerably. Examples of open kinetic chain exercises are; bicep curl, lateral raise, leg extension and pectoral flye.

Closed kinetic chain exercises are described as an exercise where the hands or feet are fixed against an immoveable object (usually the floor) and the body moves to and from the point of contact. Closed kinetic chain exercises are of a compound (multi-joint exercises) nature and are considered safer than open kinetic chain exercises, as the increase of resistance is added to the body (core), and therefore reducing the stress on a single joint or muscle.

Sports therapists and coaches both agree that closed kinetic chain exercises are better for you than open kinetic chain exercises due to their functional day to day compound movements and representation of sporting activities, however, open chain exercises and isolation movements do have their benefits and are still very appropriate, and therefore used commonly.

Dose-response

The dose-response effect is a continuum of benefits gained through increased exercise duration, volume and intensity, and simply put, the more exercise we participate in, and at a higher intensity, the greater the fitness gains. However, as you may be aware, our fitness level does have a limit, and if it didn't we could all potentially become super-humans, so in respect of this, at a particular point, the benefits begin to taper off and plateau, this is usually around 60 minutes, and the highest degree of benefits gained are around 30-60 minutes. This does not mean that after 60 minutes you gain no further benefits, you do, they are just not so obvious or tangible. Training beyond 60 minutes offers massive benefits to an endurance athlete, not only physically but also psychologically.

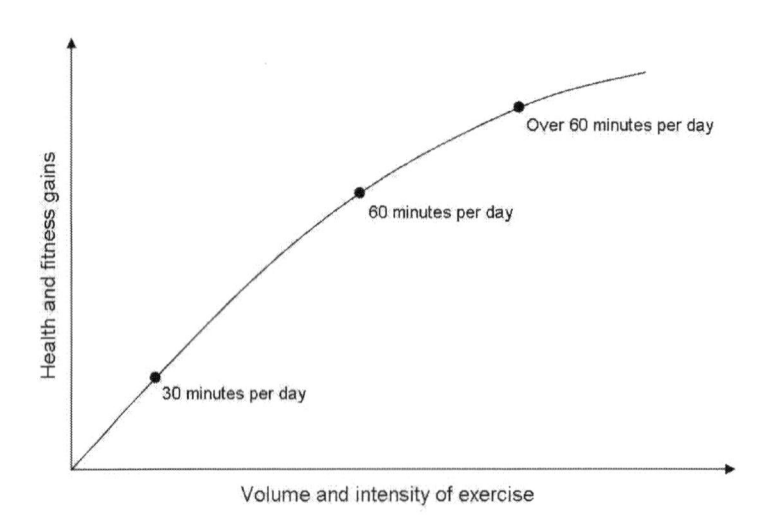

Many studies have been conducted into the dose-response relationship, and exact guidelines of the benefits are unclear. The above diagram is a visual guide to demonstrate how benefits taper off as more time and intensity are introduced, therefore we must take into consideration that everybody is different and benefits gained are going to be very individual to that person.

Overtraining

If you are a serious weight trainer or you regularly participate in exercise, you may be aware of how obsessed you can become, maybe you aren't aware, and actually that's where the problem of overtraining and overtraining syndrome may occur. There is a theory that this addiction to exercise is due to the endorphins and dopamine which are generated during exercise (and other enjoyable activities!) Regular fitness training has multiple benefits to our health and fitness; we are constantly reminded of how we should all be exercising to reap these benefits. However, it is as equally important to ensure that we are not doing too much, and often we can be blinded by the motivation and feel good factor that working out brings.

Overtraining is the principle of doing too much and not having enough rest between sessions, it can be easily avoided if you follow the correct training regime, but if it does start to occur, you may begin to experience some of the following symptoms; and that's when you know it might be time to adjust your training. Illness (including regular colds) due to a suppressed immune system, de-motivation and lack of interest to exercise, susceptibility to injury and/or longer term recovery, depression and inability to sleep, a plateau in your training and even reversibility.
Remember, your body recovers and rebuilds during rest, and the amount of rest needs to be adequate for the amount of stress induced during training, in other words, even if you are having rest, if it is not enough in order to recover from the training, then overtraining will occur. So it is really important that you recognise this and allow yourself rest days from the gym. You can always have active rest too, doing some kind of activity that is not related to you main training.
Overtraining syndrome is more common and usually occurs in weight trainers, but it is also a threat to runners and other athletes.

Delayed onset muscle soreness (DOMS)

DOMS is described as the pain and soreness felt 2-3 days after intense exercise. You are most likely to feel this soreness if you have increased the intensity of your programme, have not been exercising for a while, are new to exercise or trying something new. DOMS is part of an adaptation process to a training stimulus, and many people (particularly beginners to exercise) may find this response disturbing, negative and unpleasant, of course it is unpleasant; however, it is a sure way of increasing strength and muscle size (hypertrophy). Negative, or eccentric training (muscle lengthens under tension) is most associated with DOMS, this will cause the most soreness and is thought to be caused by microscopic tears in the muscle. The severity of tearing and the soreness will be related to and dependant on the amount of stress placed upon the muscle.

DOMS is not the fatigue or pain felt during or immediately after exercise, and as the name suggests, it is a delayed response, usually at its worse 48 hours post exercise. The pain is often described as sensitive to touch and dense, and many exercisers complain the day after a session they have DOMS, no, they don't, and they often need to work much harder in order to experience it!

It is commonly believed that stretching will prevent post exercise muscle soreness and DOMS, there has been no proven evidence to suggest this, and other studies have been conducted to prove otherwise.

So we cannot avoid the onset of DOMS if we have exercised hard or introduced an unfamiliar exercise, it is going to happen and therefore unavoidable, however, there are a few thing you could try to help reduce and relieve the symptoms, they will not all work for everyone, so try them out next time and see what works for you.

Gentle stretching
Try some gentle stretching after you session, particularly around the areas and muscles worked. Be sure not to put too much stress on the muscle and make things worse.

Massage
Massaging the area can help to flush out toxins from the muscle and help improve circulation; this in turn will ensure adequate nutrients are being delivered to the muscles.

Ice bath
Some people swear by this treatment, it is often spoken about in regards to post treatment following a long run, but is also a regular routine for most professional rugby players and elite athletes. The immense cold of the ice water (12-15 degrees Celsius) is thought to constrict blood vessels and therefore reduce swelling.

Anti-inflammatory
Not highly recommended as the pain reliever leaves you unaware of potential problems occurring (during an activity), so therefore after exercise would be more suitable to help reduce any inflammation.

R.I.C.E
Consider the usual rest, ice, compression and elevation treatment that is recommended for sprains and strains; however it might prove awkward to elevate numerous areas of the body at the same time. Compression tights (and arm tights) are worn by many as a way of reducing swelling in the arms and legs during and after exercise.

Monitoring intensity

Whether you are training a client or training yourself, you need to have some way of monitoring the intensity that you are working at, for the reasons of ensuring the effectiveness of the exercise and also to give you something to work towards; a goal in relation to the intensity. There are many ways in which you can do this, and the mode you chose will be determined and affected by many factors; including, training on your own, equipment available and environment. You decide which mode suites you and your client the best, and remember more than one approach can be used at the same time to ensure effective monitoring.

Heart rate

We have two ways in which we can use heart rate to monitor intensity, max heart rate or the heart rate reserve method, known as the Karvonen formula.
In order to use the max heart rate method, you need to work out your max heart rate by doing the below calculation. Once you have done

this, you then need to calculate the percentage of MHR you want to work at.

220 – 30(age) = 190bpm (max heart rate)

70% = 190(MHR) x 0.7 = 133bpm
80% = 190(MHR) x 0.8 = 152bpm
90% = 190(MHR) x 0.9 = 171bpm

This is a very general way in which to use heart rate as a way of monitoring intensity, but what it doesn't take into consideration is, an individual's fitness level, it assumes that all people of the same age are able to work at the same intensity.

Heart rate reserve method is a much more accurate way of calculating the percentage of max heart rate, unlike the above example; this method uses the difference between some ones maximum heart rate and their resting heart rate. You use the 220 – age formula to calculate max heart rate and you also need to measure resting heart rate, this is best done first thing in the morning after a good night of sleep; measure it over a few days and take the average. Once you have done this you can use the calculation below.

Max heart rate = 190
Resting heart rate = 60

190(MHR) – 60(RHR) resting heart rate = 130(HRR) heart rate reserve

70% = 130(HRR) x 0.7 = 91 + 60(RHR) = 151bpm
80% = 130(HRR) x 0.8 = 104 + 60(RHR) = 164bpm
90% = 130(HRR) x 0.9 = 117 + 60(RHR) = 177bpm

The advantage of using heart rate reserve is that it allows a fitter individual to work at a higher BPM of heart rate compared to a less fit person, whilst at the same heart rate percentage. This is based on the assumption that the fitter we are, the lower the resting heart rate we have, and the lower the resting heart rate, the higher the intensity we can work at. However, do be aware that some people have naturally low resting heart rates which may not be related to fitness, and also certain medication can cause lower resting heart rates.

If you are working from a gym, you'll have the added bonus of heart rate sensors on the cardiovascular machines, if you're working outside of a gym then you will need to use a heart rate monitor, and without either of these you will have to opt for another way of monitoring intensity.

Heart rate training zones

Using heart rate to monitor intensity can be a really effective way of training, and a good understanding of the different training zones and how to calculate your clients' heart rate is vital. The different training zones offer different physiological benefits, and when prescribing CV exercise, knowing your clients goals and fitness level is really important in order to achieve this.
The below information is a guide only and these guidelines may not suit everyone, nor be a truly accurate way of determining intensity.

Moderate or fat burning zone 55-70% MHR
This is a great place to start for beginners to exercise, it offers health benefits, and some clients may even see improvements to their fitness. Being called the fat burning zone can often be misleading, clients wanting to reduce body fat will stay at this low level, believing they will burn lots of fat. In this zone, the intensity is low, and therefore so is the overall amount of calories used, however, the percentage of calories used from fat when working at this level is high in proportion to the percentage of glucose.

Fitness zone 70-80% MHR
Improvements to fitness for most people begin in the fitness zone, such as higher stroke volume, increased VO2 max and increased lung capacity. Adaptations such as improved aerobic glycolysis and oxygen transportation will enable the exerciser to work at a higher level than before.

Aerobic performance zone 80-90% MHR
The benefits of the fitness zone will also be achieved at this level of heart rate and intensity; also, aerobic and anaerobic thresholds will increase at this level (this is the point in which blood lactate levels rise to the point of 2 and 4mmoLs respectively), therefore increasing

aerobic capacity by delaying the onset and improving how the body flushes it away.

Anaerobic performance zone 90-100% MHR

Working continuously at this level of intensity for extended periods of time is just not possible; therefore, interval training is an ideal way of doing so; for example, experiencing the intensity for short periods of time followed by a longer rest, and sprint intervals would be a perfect example of this. Improvements in VO2 max and increased anaerobic enzymes are the main benefits of training in this zone, as well as improved type 2b muscle fibre recruitment.

Onset blood lactate accumulation (OBLA)

During aerobic exercise, blood lactate levels increase, and as long as the intensity (and therefore blood lactate levels) do not rise, the circulatory system can easily deal with and flush away this lactate. This is referred to as the aerobic threshold, and at the point in which blood lactate levels reach 2mmols. If intensity does increase, and therefore blood lactate levels rise, the muscle may begin to experience a burning sensation and major fatigue, this would be a clear indication that you have reached your anaerobic threshold and muscle contraction becomes compromised as blood lactate levels reach 4mmols, at this level, blood lactate is being produced quicker than it can be flushed away.

Borg scale 6-20 and RPE

The Borg scale was originally devised using twenty year old students as the subjects and is related to heart rate of this age group. Two hundred and twenty (the figure to calculate max heart rate) minus 20 (the age of the students) leaves you with two hundred, an average resting heart rate is sixty beats per minute, so this 60 to 200 became the numbers used for this alternative method of monitoring intensity, 6 being no effort at all and 20 being maximum effort.

RPE	Heart Rate (bpm)	Description
6	60	No effort
7	70	Very very light
8	80	
9	90	Very light
10	100	
11	110	Light intensity
12	120	
13	130	Slightly hard
14	140	
15	150	Hard
16	160	
17	170	Very hard
18	180	
19	190	Near maximum
20	200	Maximum, very intense

As you can see, the Borg scale relates to the given intensity, for example; 20 (or 200) sits with 100% MHR, and in a 20 year old 100% of MHR equals 200bpm. This may sound a little confusing at first, but don't worry, because when using the Borg scale to monitor intensity our clients are working at, we simply use the numbers and descriptions related to them, because let's face it, not all of our clients are going to be twenty years old!

The Borg scale is a great tool for monitoring intensity, but you might agree that the numbers from six to twenty are difficult to relate to how hard you feel you are working. Try this exercise; give me a number from 6-20 based on how happy you're feeling right now, six being the unhappiest you have ever been and twenty the happiest and you couldn't imagine being happier. I guess you did ok using this scale but it's not the easiest to use is it? Hopefully you are all happy though. The ACSM (American College of Sports Medicine) developed a much easier scale from 1-10 called the rate of perceived exertion (RPE) or how it feels scale. This, as it suggests, it uses a much easier 1-10 scale as opposed to 6-20, see the diagram below.

1	Very, very light – no effort
2	Very easy – slight effort
3	
4	Moderate – slightly breathless
5	
6	Fairly hard – quite breathless
7	
8	Very hard – intense
9	
10	Maximum effort – very intense

If you have already completed some or all of your fitness qualifications, you would have already been introduced to both of these scales. You would have been encouraged to use the Borg scale, but in reality you are unlikely to use it with clients and have probably already decided that the 1-10 scale is more useful. Once you get familiar with the scale yourself, you will no longer feel the need to have it on paper and consistently throw it in your clients face and ask them how they are feeling every single minute.

As you become more experienced at teaching, you will become an expert at monitoring intensity and learn to use a verbal version of the 1-10 scale along with many other methods to check that your client is working at the appropriate level, therefore and most importantly you will get an effective workout.

Talk test

The talk test is a very useful and effective way to monitor your client whilst they are exercising. Simply by talking to your client, you can get a very accurate indicator of intensity. Of course it does require your client to talk to you, and it is while they talk you get to see how hard they are working. For the average person, walking slow should be no effort and having a conversation at the same time should be no problem. Increase the pace to a brisk walk and you may start to feel your heart beat a little faster, get a little warmer and feel slightly breathless, but you may still feel able to hold a conversation without puffing too much. Take this into a run and your ability to talk will undoubtedly become harder as you have to pause between words to catch a breath. The talk test works excellently in conjunction with a 1-10 or 6-20 RPE chart. Using the talk test shouldn't really be something you tell your client about just before you use it, I mean you don't want to explain to your client how you are going to use it, just in case they somehow use it to their advantage and make their session easier!

Calories

Many people are obsessed with counting calories, and this can often be the case when using cardiovascular machines. Most CV equipment will display the amount of calories burnt and some people like to use this as a way of monitoring what they are doing. In my experience, this is not an effective way of monitoring intensity, but it does help to keep the client motivated, and allows them to tell their friends how many calories they burned at the gym! Total calories burnt, does not monitor intensity, but the machine may also display calories per hour, which is way more effective because it relates to the intensity they are working at there and then. For example; if you are on the rowing machine and the console displays one hundred calories per hour, and then you pick up the pace, the calories per hour may increase to one hundred and twenty calories per hour, indicating a higher level of intensity. This way of monitoring is not the most common but can still be effective.

METs

MET stands for metabolic equivalent of task, and relates to metabolism and calories. Even at complete rest we are still using energy and burning calories, this is known as our basal metabolic rate or BMR, everybody is different and we all have different BMRs. As far as using this as an intensity indicator, somebody's BMR would be equal to the number one, so if you were to work at a level that was twice the effort and therefore burning twice the amount of calories this would be at a level of 2 METs. If the level was ten times the intensity and burning ten times the calories of someone's BMR, then they would be working at a level of 10 METs.

When recording the total MET's after a period of exercise, multiply the number of minutes spent exercising by the MET level, for example:

Working for 25 minutes at a level of 6 MET's (25 x 6) = 150 MET's

Chapter 7

Information gathering, programming and training

Your main role as a personal trainer is to write programmes and deliver exercise sessions, however, the difference between doing this as a gym instructor and personal trainer is that the programme is very specific to the client and you work with this person on a regular basis. You have to draw on your experience and the technical knowledge you have learnt in order to manage and deliver effective training sessions. As a gym instructor, you may still write appropriate programmes for people, but these programmes are left for the client to follow alone, and sometimes, a 'one size fits all' approach is used by gym instructors. I must admit that during my time as a gym instructor I wrote many programmes for people that may have been almost identical, but then one of the reasons I went on to personal training was to work more individually with people.

In order to write programmes for people that are specific to them, it is really important that we ensure we gather enough relevant information, for example; just finding out about their goals is nowhere near enough information, ok so you might find out what they want, but they have barriers (everyone has barriers to exercise, everyone!), this is where our advanced skills come into play as we begin to establish important information about our client that will allow us to tailor the exercise regime exactly to them.

Below is an extensive list of things to find out about your client before you can start to write them a programme. Some of this information may seem obvious to gather, but I have included it anyway.

Personal details

Description of lifestyle

Occupation

Past and current activity levels

Goals (SMART) and needs

Exercise likes and dislikes

Barriers to exercise

Time available

Stage of change

Reason/motivation to change

Health/medical conditions/injuries

Where to train

With this information gathered during the consultation, you should then be able to design an exercise regime for you client. One more piece of information that you may need to gather which could either be done as part of the consultation or during the first session is some fitness testing; but remember, the fitness tests that you decide to deliver must be specific to their goals, however, doing one or two tests that are not specific to their goals may actually highlight something that the client needs to work on but wasn't actually aware of, this is a client need, they may know what they want or don't want, but they will usually be unaware of what they actually need.

When it comes to programme prescription, it is useful to use the FITT principle, this stands for Frequency (how many times per week), Intensity (how hard and what level), Time (amount of time spent per session) and Type (what kind of exercise). This is very useful tool that can be used to give an overview of your clients' regime over a period of weeks, helping you to write more specific individual training programmes.

Working with different client groups

You will be faced working with different groups of people throughout your fitness career, and these different groups of people are sometimes referred to as special populations, but personally I do like this term, everybody is different and unique, and therefore we shouldn't categorize people, but rather consider their needs individually. That said, with different client groups, we must be aware that they all have different needs and therefore different considerations need to be made. The following guidelines are not to be taken literally, as people from these different groups can have varying fitness levels and abilities, and as I remember, a colleague of mine always said, "We shouldn't wrap these people up in cotton wool!"

It is important to mention at this stage, that if you are planning on offering your services to any of these groups of people, you must ensure you have a valid qualification, not just for legal reasons, but also for the health and safety of the individual. The content in this section is by no means comprehensive, nor can it be considered evidence of formal training, it is merely a guide to give you an idea of what to consider.
It might be that if you are working in a gym and someone who fits into one of these groups comes in for an induction, then you have some skills and knowledge to see them through the session, but what we shouldn't be doing is writing programmes and training these people on a regular basis without specialist knowledge.

Older adults

The title older adults, is not an ideal term used for this group of people, particularly when you consider that's what you are at 50+. Some of my friends and colleagues are of this age group and are some of the fittest people I know, but we cannot deny nature and the fact that our bodies begin to deteriorate around our thirties, and therefore, in some people, by the time they are 50 nature has taken a crash course on them and this process is well underway.
We all know by eating well, controlling stress levels and partaking in physical activity and exercise that we can delay this process but eventually it will happen to all of us.

Considerations

Bones become weaker and less dense, increasing the likelihood of breaks and fractures. Neuromuscular pathways break down and become less effective. Articular cartilage wears out, causing bone to rub on bone within synovial joints and causing osteoarthritis, and more importantly pain.

- Increased susceptibility to fractures
- Less stability and ROM around joints
- Reduced shock absorbency
- Increased blood pressure
- Decreased efficiency of circulation

What to prescribe

- Functional activities
- Multi joint exercises
- Core stability
- Motor skills

What to avoid

- High impact
- Spinal flexion
- Complex exercises

One of the most important types of exercise for older adults is weight bearing exercise, particularly post menstrual women; this means, exercises that puts stress on muscles and their attaching site to the bone. This pulling of muscle on bone encourages the process of bone density, and this can help reduce the risk of breaks and fractures.

Teenagers and children

When working with teenagers and children, there are two things you must consider; they are still growing and their bones in particular are susceptible to fractures if too much force is placed on the muscle.
This could potentially stunt their growth by damaging the epiphyseal plate in their bones; this is the site of growth within a long bone. The other point to consider is that although they have a very effective

cardiovascular system for their size compared to an adult, they are at risk of overheating during prolonged intense aerobic exercise because their ability to cool themselves down has not yet fully developed; and younger children have an inability to sweat, which is a way of the body cooling itself down.

Considerations

- Implications of the incomplete fusing of the epiphyseal plates
- Tight muscles due to bone growth.
- Susceptible to overheating

What to prescribe

- Body weight exercises
- Functional activities (pushing/pulling)
- Development of motor skills
- Interval based CV training

What to avoid

- High intensity strength training
- Prolonged high intensity CV training

Ante/post natal

Considerations

During pregnancy and for a period after, the hormone relaxin is produced and released from the placenta and the ovaries. This hormone is responsible for relaxing ligaments in the pelvis, and so joint stability is compromised. There are also circulation concerns for mother and baby after the first trimester, the concern is that the weight of the baby can sit on and cut off circulation to mother and baby, so therefore certain exercise positions should be avoided.
Mother and baby are also at risk of overheating during exercise.

- Reduced stability around joints
- Increased joint range of movement

- Change in centre of gravity (balance)
- Change of posture
- Overheating

What to prescribe

- Interval type exercise
- Maintenance stretches (not developmental)
- Core stability
- Balance exercises

What to avoid

- Supine (lying on back) after 1st trimester
- Developmental stretches
- High impact exercise

Disabled clients

When dealing with people with disabilities it is really important to treat each disability individually, there are many forms of mental and physical disability, and therefore way too much information to go into this book. If you happen to train someone with any disability, it would be very wise to do some research beforehand, giving you a general idea of the condition and how it can affect exercise, and also how exercise can affect the disability. Doing this research before you meet your client will show great customer care and professionalism towards your client. It is also really important to discuss the condition with your client, find out from them what they can and can't do, after all, they're the one with the disability. Perhaps their condition is so severe that they require a carer; and therefore you have to liaise with them in order to communicate. Working with disabled people can be challenging, but at the same time it can be very rewarding and usually a good working relationship is built.

SMART goal setting

The purpose of this section is to give you a basic understanding of progressive programming, helping you to identify clients' goals and needs, therefore enabling you to write an effective training programme.
One of the roles of a personal trainer is to deliver effective exercises, and in order to do that you need to have a plan, a plan that consists of what it is you are going to be delivering in order to help your clients achieve their goals.
The most important factor to consider when writing your client a programme is to identify what it is that your client actually wants to achieve from their fitness regime. A lot of the time when you ask a client what they want to achieve they are very likely to say something like, "I want to get fitter", "I want to be stronger" or "I want to lose weight", these are a few of the most common client goals, well actually to me these are not goals at all, these are client 'wants', they are just statements, and most importantly, we as personal trainers cannot help someone effectively if they give us very broad statements as I have just given you. I want you to do a very quick exercise for me, I want you imagine you are a personal trainer (apologies if you are already, but do it anyway) and sitting with a client during a consultation, choose one of my common statements from above and ask yourself whether you think you have gathered enough information from this imaginary client in order to allow you to write them an effective programme?
There is much information to gather during a client consultation which we will cover shortly, but based merely on what the client wants to achieve, do you really feel confident to design a workout/programme? Have a think about it for a moment and come back to reading once you have done so.
If you did complete the exercise, welcome back and well done! Hopefully your answer was something like 'no that is not enough information and is not very specific', if that's the case then you are absolutely right; these common goals are not SMART.

S stands for specific, and goals have to be specific, let me use one of my examples from earlier; the 'I want to get fitter' goal is a good one to use. Firstly I would ask "what does fitness mean?" as you may know there are five components of physical fitness, these are;

cardiovascular fitness, muscular strength, muscular endurance, flexibility and motor fitness (skills). So you would ask yourself, or more importantly your client, what area of fitness did they want to improve, this is where you may have to educate your client to a degree on these different areas. Sometimes asking "what does being fit mean to you?" can provoke your client into telling you exactly what they would like to be able to do, once they do this, you can then identify which area of fitness they need to work on. For example, if your client says "I want to be able to climb the stairs without getting breathless" you'll realise they actually want to improve their cardiovascular fitness.

Most of the time people won't have specific goals, and you'll have to work with them in order to establish some, however, sometimes they will have very specific goals, and a common example of this would be someone who wanted to run in a 10k race, this can make the whole process so much easier, but there is still more work to do!

I often use the saying 'if you don't know where you're going, then how are you going to know when you get there?' you can use that one for free if you like!

Perhaps your client wants to run the full 10k because last time they walked half of it and only ran 5k, so always discuss some of the finer details of their goal.

The **M** in SMART stands for measureable; the clients goal needs to be measureable, how else are you going to know when the goal has been achieved? In the 10k example this is already done for you, and it is measureable because the race and distance is 10k, that's 10,000 metres or about 6.25 miles in case you're unfamiliar. But when someone says that they want to get fitter, or in the example used to increase cardiovascular fitness because they want to be able to climb stairs, you need to establish and agree to what level of fitness they want to achieve.

So we know that our client wants to improve their cardiovascular fitness, but they do not have any specific goals and are not doing any sporting events. So what can we suggest to the client? We need to give this goal a measureable aspect, because although we have established improving cardiovascular fitness, it is not measureable. What you may want to do are some fitness tests to establish 'where they are at' right now. May I suggest that if 'climbing stairs without getting puffed' is your clients' goal, then test them on their ability to climb stairs in a set period of time or to complete a certain number in the fastest time, this way you'll benchmark their cardiovascular fitness based on exactly what they have identified to achieve, and this will also help to keep them motivated.

With this information gathered you can then both decide on an improvement (goal). Let us pretend that during your clients' fitness test of climbing stairs they managed to climb 200 steps in 2 minutes 35 seconds, you could set them a goal of achieving the same number of steps in 2 minutes 20 seconds.

So now we need to discuss the **A** of SMART, this stands for achievable, is the goal that you have set achievable? And is your client capable of reaching that goal. This is where you must be realistic and honest with your client, because sometimes clients may just suggest a goal that is not going to be attainable. Let me tell you about a goal setting experience I had with a client during my time as a gym instructor, I had an induction with a lady who had a clear goal of losing weight. This particular lady was in her mid-forties, and her goal was to get down to a weight of eleven stone, yes get 'back' to eleven stone, so she has been there before which is half the battle and a massive advantage to achieving goals, I proceeded to ask her 'when' she was this weight, she replied "when I was twenty one!". Obviously the issue here is the fact that twenty one was a good twenty years ago and as we age our bodies change, particularly more in females. I then had to spend the next five minutes with her explaining the physiological reasons why this was a big ask and very unlikely to be achieved without starving herself and compromising her health. You have to be honest with your clients, tactfully tell them whether their goal is a pipedream or not. Over time as a personal trainer you will become familiar with what is achievable and what is not for different client groups.

The key to setting measurable targets is to always underestimate what your client is likely to achieve, consider this example; if you came to me for personal training and said you wanted to increase your muscle mass by 10%, I may suggest that we start off by setting a target of 5%, this will obviously be more achievable and when this happens you will be motivated knowing you have achieved the goal we set. However, if we stuck with your initial 10% goal and were unable to achieve it, that would not be motivating at all, even to the point of you thinking, I wasn't a very effective personal trainer.

And now the **R** in SMART; this stands for realistic. Achievable and realistic are going to appear very similar indeed, but let me explain the R, and you can make your own mind up. We just looked at achievable, and whether someone would actually be able to get the results they wanted, in the example we just used this was a 5% increase in muscle mass, based on the information gathered and after further discussions with your client, you have decided that this is definitely doable. The only problem is now; actually getting to the gym, finding the time and the motivation to do it. Let us assume that you live far away from a gym and do not drive, you have a really busy schedule with work and family life and no one to train with, which has a massive impact on your motivation. What we have just identified are some very realistic and common barriers in which people face, and if these barriers are unavoidable or cannot be overcome at all, the realism of achieving the goal set becomes unrealistic.

We need to do some lifestyle investigation to identify whether the client is able to achieve their goal, it might be achievable if we drag it out over a very long period of time, but let's face it; some people want results in minimal time these days, due to the busy nature of life in the twenty first century.

This then leads us nicely to the **T** in SMART, and this stands for timed. It is all good and well having a specific, measurable, achievable and realistic goal if you are not going to put a time on it, what this means is you have to set a target time, the 10k runner wants to run the full 10k buy June 10th next year, the 5% muscle mass increase wants to be achieved in 12 weeks, and the stair climber wants to achieve their 220 steps in 2 minutes in 6 weeks time. If we never set a time or date target then it just gives the client an eternity to reach their goals, and this isn't going to help anyone. Try and think back to the last time you had to do something by a certain date or time and remember how motivated or maybe stressed you felt in order to get it done. Now I'm not suggesting we encourage our clients to feel stressed about reaching their goals in a set time, but it will certainly keep them on their feet with the thought of running out of time before they reach their goal. If you're lucky, they may even over achieve their goal, and if this happens, you have a client that is achieving their goals, remaining motivated, and loving their fantastic personal trainer!

Hopefully now you understand the importance of setting goals, or more importantly SMART goals. It will help you to write an effective programme, deliver effective training sessions and keep track of what your client is doing, allowing to also monitor progress, it will also help to keep your client motivated and feeling involved in their fitness.

You may want to consider setting your client medium and short term goals if their long term goal is a long way off. This will help to keep your client motivated and constantly reminded what they are working towards. You must also set review points, for which you are going to assess your client and identify whether the set goals are being achieved.

Barriers to exercise

Everybody has barriers, and especially barriers to exercise, think about it for a moment; if exercise barriers didn't exist then everybody would be exercising, and the reason why everyone is not exercising is because they have barriers, simple.

As a personal trainer it will be your job to identify barriers that your client may have and not actually be aware of. As your communication skills improve and you gain more experience of doing the job, this task will become a whole lot easier. It's very useful to identify and record your client's barriers to exercise, your next job will be to discuss these barriers with your client and together come up with appropriate strategies to help reduce or completely overcome them.

Finding the right weight

When you enter the gym or begin training your client at home for the first time, one of the first things you will be faced with doing is assessing what your client is capable of. It would be assumed that at this point you will know if your client is a beginner, familiar with exercise or a regular exerciser from the information you gathered during the consultation. You may have also performed some fitness assessments to determine their current fitness level. If your client is a beginner, you are most likely to have to demonstrate the exercises you want your client to perform, even if they think they know how to do it, it would certainly be a good idea to do this in order for them to see how the exercise should be performed properly, and this is why as a personal trainer your technique has to be perfect. Sometimes a silent demo may be appropriate, but only if the exercise is so complex and you think 'just watching' is appropriate. Remember, a picture paints a thousand words, and if your client can see it, they are more likely to understand it. With all this in mind, and an exercise plan in place, you are ready to begin training your client.

The first task for you as the trainer is to find the correct weight or resistance for them. When getting your client to perform the exercise for the first time, it is really important that the resistance is minimal; this is to ensure your client can initially perform the exercise with correct technique, loading up the weight and performing with incorrect technique will increase the risk of injury and depending on the exercise can lead to poor posture. Once you are happy with technique and it has been performed enough times correctly, it is now time to increase the weight. Finding the correct weight for your client is a process of trial and error and may take a bit of time to establish.

It would be a wise idea to select a weight that your client is likely to be able to lift than that of one that might be a little over ambitious. If you select a weight that is too heavy, then the client may feel disappointed and de-motivated at the fact that they cannot lift the given weight, whereas, if give them a weight that they are more likely to achieve, then this will have the opposite effect, giving them the confidence and motivation they need to carry on and progress.

If you are instructing an experienced or advanced client, the way you go about assessing the appropriate weight is a little different. To start with, there is likely to be less need for a demonstration if the client tells you that they have performed the exercise before, however, sometimes a client might need a recap of the exercise, and in this case a quick demonstration is needed, but not a lengthy one. It is usually a good idea to ask your experienced exerciser to show you the exercise and how they perform it, by doing this you can check technique and reinforce teaching points, and of course identify whether they are doing it correctly, and more importantly identify whether or not they need a proper demonstration. Even experienced exercises sometimes perform exercises with bad technique, and just because someone has been exercising for a long time, it certainly doesn't mean they are doing it correctly.

Once good technique is established with your experienced exerciser it is time to start piling on the weight, but before you do this it would be very beneficial to ask them what kind of weight they usually lift for the exercise, and by doing this you will be much closer to identifying the appropriate weight much sooner. The trial and error approach applies to the experienced exerciser too, however, you are more likely to find it easier and quicker, saving time, and giving your client more exercise for their money.

Whether your client is a beginner or advanced exerciser, it is important to let them know the repetition range they are working with in order to establish the correct weight, and it goes without saying that the number of repetitions you prescribe should relate to their goals. Constantly reminding your client how many repetitions they are aiming for (as they perform the exercise) can really help them to establish the correct weight and keep them motivated.

Resistance training approaches

In this section we are going to explore a whole range of different resistance training approaches that you can either use yourself for your own training, or to use with your clients and incorporate them into their programme.

Before we get started, and so you can clearly understand these training approaches to their maximum potential, we need to discuss something called the muscular strength and endurance continuum.

⎯⎯⎯⎯⎯⎯⎯⎯⎯⎯⎯⎯⎯⎯⎯⎯⎯⎯⎯⎯⎯⎯⎯⎯⎯➤

Strength   Endurance
1 repetition   25 repetitions

Take a look at the diagram, on one end we have strength and on the other end we have endurance. We are talking 'muscular' strength and endurance here, that is of most importance.
It will be a good idea at this stage to identify the definitions of muscular strength and muscular endurance.

Muscular strength is defined as the maximum amount of resistance or force a muscle or group of muscles can overcome once; otherwise known as a 1RM (one repetition maximum), and a repetition maximum is just that, you cannot do 2, not even for a million pounds (well maybe that would motivate some people to do another one, but I think you get the idea), this would be a physical demonstration of pure strength.

Muscular endurance on the other hand is a little different, and endurance means to last a longer period of time, so therefore muscular endurance is the ability of a muscle or group of muscles to overcome a sub-maximal resistance over a prolonged period of time, and therefore many repetitions. On the diagram you may notice we have only gone up to 25 repetitions, this isn't a definitive cut off point to gain the benefits of endurance training, it just means that if we start going beyond this amount of repetitions then we start to enter the realms of cardiovascular fitness, and here the benefits differ to that of resistance training.

When prescribing resistance training an important aspect to consider is overload if the approaches selected are to be effective. Some people think that overload is a bad thing, actually it isn't bad at all, it is a positive thing, and it basically means doing more than what you are accustomed to, just pushing yourself that little bit further. If you do not apply overload to your training approach you will not reap the benefits of the approach.

A beginner to exercise may only have to apply a small amount of overload, as they are not used to pushing themselves, nor are they familiar with how they should feel, the focus should be on just 'feeling it' perhaps, slight fatigue maybe. You will also consider the approach you would prescribe a beginner as some are very advanced training systems and will be unsuitable and potentially unsafe for beginners. Remember, if you push a beginner too hard and prescribe advanced training approaches, then they may decide to not come back!

On the other hand, an experienced weight trainer may be very used to working to a very high intensity and advanced training approaches.

The following training approaches have been designed by researchers and weight trainers to give you the best possible results from your training. All of these training approaches have different benefits when performed correctly, so knowing your clients resistance training goals is of most importance to ensure the correct training approach has been selected. I have indicated who they may be most suitable for as they vary in difficulty and intensity.

Single set training

This is the most simple and essentially the most effective type of resistance training. Only one set of a given number of repetitions is performed before moving on to another exercise, for example; 1 set of 15 repetitions. This is where everybody will begin; it is the starting point for resistance training. Although it is a very straight forward way of training, many experienced weight lifters will still use this type of training to compliment their already advanced regime.

Basic sets

Basic sets is exactly the same as the above approach, the only difference is that after the first set and after a short rest, you then perform another set. Essentially, you can perform as many sets as you like, the only limiting factor will be energy used and fatigue in the muscles involved.

Circuit approach

Here we have an approach that comprises of multiple exercises and all performed using a single set training approach. A circuit approach is performed in exactly the same way you would expect a regular circuit class to be performed. Most people will do this type of approach without even realising it. All you need to do here is select a series of exercises, perform one set and move on to the next once each exercise has been completed. You may perform this circuit more than once and as many times as you like. This is a great way of exercising and particularly good for beginners and less experienced exercises. One of the benefits is that you won't overtire any particular muscle as long as you chose a mix of different body parts for your circuit. There is a short rest in between exercises as you move from one to the other, however, although you can chose a rest time between exercises (usually the time it takes to get to the next exercise) your heart will have to work hard to pump blood all around the body and to the different areas you are working, therefore, a circuit approach will also give you a fantastic aerobic workout which will result in further fat loss.

Supersets

Supersets are essentially two exercises performed back to back with no rest in between. Obviously there will be a very short period of time between the two exercises, but this must be as little as possible. Supersets can be performed in two distinctive ways. Firstly, the exercises/muscles selected must oppose each other, so for example; quadriceps and hamstrings, leg extension followed by seated leg curl. By doing this, you can go straight to another exercise with no rest, and that is because you are working completely different muscles.
The second way of performing this approach is by selecting exercises that target the same muscles of the body. An easy way to do this might be to chose two pushing exercises or two pulling exercises, for example, a bent over row followed by the lat pulldown machine, both exercises primarily work the latissimus dorsi and biceps. Performing two similar exercises for the same area, back to back with minimal rest is going to be very challenging on the chosen area. This increases overload on the muscles, works different fibres of the muscle (as the arms will be moving in a slightly different plane) and ensures an effective workout. Increasing overload on the muscle is the main benefit of this approach, however, when choosing your repetition range for this approach, ensure you consider the doubling up of repetitions, i.e. 10 reps on each exercise will equals 20 reps in total, and 20 reps is going to give you mostly endurance benefits.

Tri-sets

This approach works in exactly the same way as supersets for the same muscle; however, you may have noticed the word tri and figured that means three! So here we have three exercises for the same area (instead of two) performed with minimal rest in between. Considerations and benefits of a tri-set are the same as a superset; it just makes it harder as you have to complete three exercises. One consideration worth thinking about is availability of equipment and not getting caught out as you're about to perform your third and final exercise (which could happen to be a fixed resistance machine) as someone decides to jump in and use that all important last machine, unless you are going to start using 'reserved' cards to attach to the machines, you may want to have a back-up plan.

Giant sets

This approach is going to be for somebody who wishes to really overload a particular area of the body. Very similar to superset same and tri-sets, a giant set relates to four or more exercises for the same muscle group, therefore muscular endurance is going to be challenged whilst gaining hypertrophy due to the high volume, particularly if this is repeated, whether that means more sets or times per week. This is a very effective and also very exhaustive approach, so consider the repetition ranges you plan to perform as you need to times that by 4, i.e. 12 repetitions x 4 exercises back to back equals 48 repetitions. Due to the nature of this approach and the fact that it works the muscle in different ways for each exercise, it would still be fair to say that you will gain some benefits relating to the repetition range of the first set, for example if my repetition range was 6, there would be significant gains in strength and hypertrophy due to the volume and endurance for the overall repetitions performed. Of course these benefits are going to be presented in varying amounts, but none the less a great approach for any experienced weight trainer, whatever their goal.

Pyramids

For an experienced exerciser wanting to gain strength and endurance benefits from their training; the pyramid approach is ideal. On a pyramid approach you chose the repetition range you want, based on your goals, but generally it will focus on strength and endurance training. The idea of this approach is to change the weight and the repetition range for each set of the same exercise. Below is a typical example of a pyramid approach.

Exercise: Lat Pull-down
1st set – 15 repetitions @ 35kg
30-60 seconds rest
2nd set – 12 repetitions @ 40kg
60-90 seconds rest
3rd set – 8 repetitions @ 45kg
90-180 seconds rest
4th set – 6 repetitions @ 50kg

A pyramid can be performed in 3 ways, the above example is an ascending pyramid, this is where the weight increases set after set. You will notice how the rest time changes, this is really dependant on your client and how prepared they are for the next set, but as the weight gets heavier a longer rest time is needed to aid short term recovery. The exact same workout can be performed but in a reverse order i.e. starting with 6 repetitions and finishing with 15 repetitions, this is known as a descending pyramid. You may chose a descending pyramid over an ascending pyramid if strength training was your goal, therefore performing the 6 repetitions from fresh and not pre-fatigued, however, it may also be beneficial to perform it as an ascending pyramid, this way you are effectively warming up the muscle or muscle groups to be worked and also by pre-fatiguing them you make the final 6 repetitions more challenging.
Finally you could go 'hard core' and perform a full pyramid, this would consist of performing an ascending pyramid and then a descending one, the above example becomes a 7 set full pyramid, not for the faint hearted or new exerciser however.

Pre and post exhaust

I have mentioned pre-fatiguing a muscle in the previous approach and how it can ensure the muscle targeted is appropriately overloaded. The pre and post exhaust approach works in exactly the same way; it does what it says on the tin, you either exhaust a muscle before or after the main exercise. The main reason why we might use this approach is to ensure the smaller muscles involved in a compound exercise are not tiring before the larger ones and therefore prohibiting an effective workout on the associated muscles. For example; if I was to perform a press up, the triceps which are the prime mover for elbow extension would usually tire before the pectoral muscles due to their smaller size, the pectorals are a large strong muscle compared to the triceps, and are generally able to produce more force. So one way around this issue is to exhaust the pectorals by means of an isolation exercise such as a dumbbell pec flye, this will tire the pectorals to a certain degree before moving on to the press up, and so in theory, during the press up, the pre exhausted pectorals should fatigue at approximately the same time as the triceps.

The post-exhaust approach is exactly the same, it just fatigues and overloads the larger muscle with an isolation exercise after the compound exercise.

Drop sets (stripping)

I have very clear memories of learning this particular resistance training approach, I was lying on the weights bench with a spotter either side of me; a spotter is someone that helps you with the weight that you may potentially struggle with, just in case you drop it on yourself! They were there either side of me as I performed a lying tricep extension, or commonly known as the 'skull crusher'. They helped to strip the bar after each set that I completed. Of course you don't have to have a spotter for this approach; it just depends on the particular exercise that you are going to do.

So the exerciser is set up to complete the first set on the chosen exercise, and usually a weight is selected that allows approximately 8-10 repetitions, but the key thing here is that you have got to be reaching near failure by the 8th to 10th repetition, otherwise the exercise is less effective. As soon as the initial set has been completed, the resistance or weight is lowered, and the amount is determined by the amount of weight first lifted, i.e. if the weight was 15kgs, it would be pointless to take it down to 5kgs for the second set, 10kgs would be the ideal choice because then you could perform a third set. However, if you have a much larger weight that you're lifting, the amount you reduce the weight by can be higher, i.e. if the first set is set at 50kgs, I could then perform the second set at 40kgs, the third at 30kgs and so on. The idea is to perform as many repetitions as possible and until failure on each set, once you have reached failure you stop, reduce the weight, and then continue to do as many repetitions as possible on the next weight without having a break in between sets. You are unlimited to the amount of times you repeat this process, 4-8 drops is about average, however, when you get to the end or your final set of this approach, you see yourself performing an average number of repetitions on a very low weight, hopefully you're not in the gym to pick someone up for a date and so they don't catch you struggling with a rather pathetic weight!

This approach demands a continuous number of repetitions over a period of time, challenging all of your energy systems and having massive benefits to you muscular endurance and hypertrophy.

Negatives

This particular approach is a favourite amongst many experienced weight trainers, and before we begin it really is an advanced approach that should only be performed by conditioned individuals and by no means by a beginner to weight training.

During a muscular contraction a muscle can either shorten or lengthen, and during the lengthening phase (eccentric) it is said we are up to about 40% stronger than the shortening phase (concentric), meaning that we are able to lift or in this case lower a heavier weight than we can lift. Imagine that someone handed you a really heavy object that was too heavy for you to keep hold of, rather than just dropping it you put the brakes on and allow the object to slowly lower to the floor, but try and lift the object from the floor and you fail because it is just too heavy to lift. In most cases as we lower a weight to the floor, the muscles that are responsible are working eccentrically (lengthening), and during this phase we are being assisted by gravity. If we attempt to lift a weight or object from the floor, then we are working against gravity, the muscles being worked have to shorten and this takes much more effort.

The scientific part of negative training is that the two protein filaments that pull against each other to bring about movement in the sarcomere within muscle fibres are actually having to detach from each other as opposed to attach as the muscle lengthens, this causes a high degree of microscopic damage to the tissue. In the short term you may wonder why you would want to do this, particularly when the soreness can be too painful to touch, and this is known as DOMS (delayed onset muscle soreness). DOMS is mostly associated with negative or eccentric training and this will usually kick in and take effect anywhere up to two days after the event, and then may last for several days, and in some cases severely restricting range of movement. However, the long term benefit is all about the strength and hypertrophy (muscle growth) gains. It is not recommended to perform this approach on the same area or muscle on consecutive workouts, and you may even avoid repeating on the same area for several days, and only after the soreness has diminished.

For this approach we will set a maximum number of eight repetitions, if you do this approach correctly you will not want or to be able to do any more than that, trust me. To start with we need to find the appropriate weight, this is the easy part, for whatever exercise we are doing, find a weight that is just a little too heavy to complete one repetition in the concentric phase, for example; a bicep curl, the concentric phase here is when you bend your elbows and lift the weight to your chest or chin; depending on how long your arms are! For the majority of exercises if you are performing a negative, then you will need a spotter, someone to help you to lift the weight, because as we've identified already, you shouldn't be able to lift the weight yourself for even one repetition. Once you have found the correct weight your spotter will help you to concentrically lift the weight, this really shouldn't be too much effort for the exerciser, so if you are the spotter then you need to ensure that you take as much of the weight as possible to avoid unnecessary fatigue. From here the exerciser will very slowly lower the weight eccentrically until the arms have straightened but not allowing the elbows to lock out.

Delorme and Watkins

This is an approach devised by Thomas L. Delorme and Arthur L. Watkins, it originated in 1945 and was referred to as 'progressive resistance exercise'. During world war two these two army physicians experimented with new rehabilitating techniques to speed up the recovery of injured servicemen.
The approach is relatively simple and offers benefits in strength for

the regular exerciser, it may not be too challenging for an experienced weight lifter, but it does allow a warm up as it progresses in weight throughout the sets. Below is an example that we can work with.

10 repetitions @ 50% of 10RM
Rest
10 repetitions @ 75% of 10RM
Rest
10 repetitions @ 100% of 10RM

This is also referred to as the 10RM system, for obvious reasons, and it does require you to find your 10RM (repetition maximum) for any given exercise, this may sometimes prove to be a little challenging. When trying to find your RM's, if too much time is spent in trial and error, then unavoidable fatigue will begin to set in, and therefore the end 10RM may not necessarily be your true 10RM weight. This may be finely tuned over a number of sessions to ensure you find your correct weight.

Once you have found your 10RM and are of course fresh; meaning not fatigued and ready to perform, then you can perform this approach. You will notice from the example above that the first set you perform is quite easy relative to the final set, and this may act as a specific warm up for your heavier sets, however, although it may be easier, it still needs to be performed with excellent technique and with a slow controlled speed. Isometric exercises are excellent for gaining strength in a specific muscle, so the slower we can execute the exercise, then the closer we can mimic this static type training. The rest period needs to be up to two minutes for maximum recovery. Perform the second set at 75% of your 10RM, and after the first set you should start to feel a degree of fatigue kick in and a hint of tiredness afterwards. Repeat the rest again for optimum recovery and then the final set. Attempting 10 repetitions of your 10RM after two sub maximal sets should really help to ensure that the final set is completely effective, and overload and failure is reached by 10 repetitions, if not before! If you feel you could have managed one more lift with a little monetary persuasion then you need to adjust and increase the weight, as this wouldn't have been your true 10RM.

Berger

In 1962, Richard Berger conducted a study on strength training, comparing single set training to multiple set training, and over a 2, 6 and 10 repetition range. From this the Berger approach was born. Three sets of six repetitions at your 6RM, this was found to give the highest increase in strength after a 12 week, 3 days per week workout period. This study was done on the bench press only, but you would hope that the benefits are exactly similar on any area of the body. The benefits you gain on multiple sets are usually less than the first set, but during the six repetition range, set three gave the highest benefit, even above the first set, and this demonstrates across the board that the 6RM range gives the highest benefits. Take a look at the table.

SETS	REPETITIONS	IMPROVEMENT
1	2	20%
2	2	17.3%
3	2	23.5%
1	6	25.5%
2	6	22.9%
3	6	29.6%
1	10	21.6%
2	10	25.1%
3	10	23%

This is a 6RM approach, so similar to the 10RM approach; a 6RM must be identified before you can execute this approach. You will have the same issues trying to find the right weight, and fatigue will set in, so ensure you find your 6RM in advance.
6 repetitions at 6RM
2-3 minutes rest
6 repetitions at 6RM
2-3 minutes rest
6 repetitions at 6RM

Due to the low repetition range, this is a strength training approach, and more rest may be necessary between sets. This approach is tough, so don't be surprised if you don't make six repetitions on the last set. Once you can complete three sets of six repetitions, it's time to retest your 6RM.

Cheat system

The cheat system is a very common approach with many experienced exercisers, and is mostly associated with free-weight exercises. This system allows the exerciser to push through the sticking phase of an exercise by either using a degree of momentum or recruiting other muscles to help initiate the exercise, this is usually through the start of the concentric phase of the exercise, for example; bending and then extending the knees to produce upward momentum whilst lifting a barbell overhead during a shoulder press. Sometimes other muscle are used to assist past this sticking point, however, the only issue with this method is that often bad technique is encouraged, and also when momentum is introduced, risk of injury increases, so therefore, the exercise should be able to be performed with good technique before the cheat system is introduced.

Using this system not only takes you past this sticking point, it also allows the associated muscles to reach an appropriate degree of overload, and usually where you would have to stop because of the sticking point and restrict the muscle, it ensures overload through a fuller range of movement.

Plyometric training

Plyometric training is a very effective form of exercise; it is sometimes referred to as SSC, which stands for Stretch Shortening Cycle. Plyometrics rely on the stretch reflex, a safety mechanism built within the nervous system; this is discussed further in types of stretching. The stretch reflex is a powerful contraction of the muscle, and this happens when there is a quick lengthening of the muscle. The quicker a muscle is stretched, the more forceful the contraction will be in response. Jumping from a box and landing on the floor produces a quick lengthening of quadriceps, glutes, gastrocnemius and soleus (as long as you bend the knees as you land), this in turn then produces a fast contraction, we then use this 'coiled' power to jump higher after we've landed. Power squats or lunges also use this same principle, if you jump in the air, land into a squat position, and from there power yourself up again, you are likely to see vast short-term improvements in height reached compared to a standard jump.

Training for power

When training for power, it is really important that you know exactly what your client wants to achieve, this is because there are many guidelines for power training, and knowing what type of power your client needs will help you to prescribe the appropriate training.
As discussed before, power is a combination of force (resistance) and velocity (speed), and to a degree, many movements and actions that we produce have some element of power, but just not very much as the resistance is far too light or we do not shift a resistance with any appropriate speed in order to call it power, so therefore, maximum power is achieved when you move a maximum resistance with maximum speed.
Power is described as either cyclic or acyclic, and the type of power required will determine the type of training. Cyclic power is a repeated powerful movement over an extended period of time, for example; a hundred metre sprinter will require cyclic power, the time to complete a hundred metre sprint is approximately ten seconds (for sprint athletes), however, the repetitions of powerful leg movements during this time is 41 if your name is Usain Bolt!
Acyclic power is a one-off bout of power, for example; a knock-out punch, shot putt or Olympic lifts. You may argue that some of these movements are done performed more than once, yes true, but a rest follows before the next takes place.
Because of the many different variables to power training, exercise prescription has to be very specific to the person and sport.

(Bompa, 1994) recommends:

8-20 repetitions
4-6 sets
50- 80% 1RM
3-5 minutes rest between sets
Performed at max speed with good technique

(Sharkey, 2002) recommends:

15-25 repetitions
30-60% 1RM
Performed at max speed with good technique
No recommendations for sets and rest between

If your sport or activity requires acyclic power, the following may be wise to consider:

1-3 repetitions
3-10 sets
90-100% 1RM
3-5 minutes rest between sets
Performed at max speed with good technique

Although there are many transferrable benefits from high repetitions with light load to low repetitions with high loads, ensuring you mimic the action of the sport (repetitions, load, and speed) is essential.

Cardiovascular training approaches

When it comes to designing your client a cardiovascular workout, you need to ensure that as well as the intensity being appropriate; so does the type of approach used.
If your client doesn't have any clear cardiovascular training goals, then using different methods may help to add variety, however, if your client does have clear goals, then choosing the correct approach and method is going to be crucial if you want to gain maximum results.

Continuous training

When it comes to improving your clients' cardiovascular (CV) fitness, you have three main approaches in which you can use. They all have their advantages and disadvantages so you need to choose the approach that is most suitable for your client, taking into consideration their goals and also their fitness level.

The most common CV approach is continuous, and this requires the exerciser to work at a set level of intensity over a prolonged period of time. This is an ideal approach for beginners as it allows them to work at a level they are comfortable with for a time period they want, it can also give a sense of achievement to the new exerciser as they may believe they are not fit enough to exercise. Although this approach is ideal for beginners, it is also a very effective approach for more experienced exercisers and clients with sports specific goals, for example; it forms a large part of your training if you are a mid to long distance runner, and as I'm sure you would agree, mid to long distance runners generally stick to a set speed throughout the race; it is very unlikely to see a long distance runner speed up and slow down unless they are in training. Consider that the average marathon time is anywhere between 2.5-4.5 hours long, that is a lot of continuous training to cope with without stopping. A disadvantage of continuous training is that it can be very monotonous and boring, even for relatively short periods of time, and clients may become easily bored.

Interval training

Interval training allows the client to work at a much higher level than usual by offering short periods of high intensity exercise followed by a lower intensity; allowing them to recover in preparation for the next burst of high intensity. A typical twenty minute interval session may consist of one minute high intensity followed by one minute recovery at a lower intensity, this cycle can then be repeated ten times, adding up to a total of twenty minutes. If you asked your client to perform for a continuous ten minutes at the given higher intensity, they would either; be unable to complete it, or complete it and not speak to you ever again! As well as allowing the client to work at a higher level of intensity, it is also a very effective approach to rapidly increase aerobic fitness because the intensity may constantly reach and challenge your clients anaerobic threshold. This is the point in which blood lactate levels reach a point where the aerobic system struggles to provide the energy we need, so the anaerobic system starts providing the majority of the energy we need, and this can usually be recognised by the burning sensation in the muscles and the extreme breathlessness.

Fartlek training

Fartlek training is usually the random programme you'll find on many CV machines. It offers a mix of high, mid and low levels of intensity for varying amounts of time. The word fartlek is Swedish, and roughly translates as 'speed play'; an approach that was specific to cross country runners experiencing changes is terrain, and therefore the level or intensity constantly changed. The ability to change the level, speed, incline and intensity on a range of cardiovascular equipment in the gym makes this approach very easy to replicate, however, because of its randomness, it is difficult to plan an exact profile of the type of session you want, unlike interval training which is very structured with set upper and lower times and intensities. The benefits of fartlek training are huge; offering those similar to interval training, but also worth considering that the varying intensities allows you to work in different heart rate training zones, this means you are using all three of your energy systems, and just like other aspects of fitness, the more you train them, the more efficient they become. Fartlek training isn't for everyone though, and I wouldn't usually give this type of approach to a beginner, it is more suited towards experienced exercisers and is very specific to some sports; in particular football and rugby. I don't want you to say you shouldn't give this approach to beginners; you just need to be aware of what is appropriate for each individual. The most appropriate way I have found to plan a fartlek session is to identify the overall time and the upper and lower limits of intensity you intend to use. Whilst training your client you have to work together to identify the level and how long to hold it for, you can then record what your client has achieved and use that to try and better it next time.

HIT (high intensity training)

High intensity training or sometimes known as HIIT (high intensity interval training) is a training concept that was devised in the seventies as a way of increasing strength and hypertrophy for weight trainers. Nowadays it is more common as a type of cardiovascular workout, and no doubt you have either participated in this type of training or have seen it on the television.

The concept is quite simple, short to medium duration of intense exercise followed by a relatively short rest period. Doesn't sound like most people's cup of tea, however the benefits are huge, the main ones being increased VO2 max and anaerobic threshold, improved glucose metabolism, an increase in strength and muscle tone and of course the aesthetic reasons of looking good! Research of this type of training has continuously identified that it utilises high levels of body fat as energy (particularly after the exercise) and the preservation of lean muscle tissue; an area of concern for many people wanting to improve cardiovascular fitness without losing lean mass.

There are many different approaches you can adopt with HIT, and Tabata interval training is a very popular example, developed by Professor Izumi Tabata; a leading sports scientist. A typical tabata consists of twenty seconds of very high intensity exercise (anaerobic, and at 170% VO2 max) followed by a ten second rest. This is repeated 8 times, and although originally performed on a cycle machine, you can either do the same exercise or change it each time, as long as the timings stay the same, see the example below.

20 seconds sprinting
10 seconds rest
20 seconds knee tucks
10 seconds rest
20 seconds burpees
10 seconds rest
20 seconds power press ups
10 seconds rest
20 seconds power lunges
10 seconds rest
20 seconds medicine ball slams
10 seconds rest
20 seconds power squats
10 seconds rest
20 seconds star jumps

Tabata intervals have been scientifically proven to give more benefits than other HIIT training programmes, even though the clinical trials had the HIIT group exercising for longer. The science behind this concept is the EPOC (excess post-exercise oxygen consumption) associated with it, and the effect it has on the body 'after' exercise, more commonly known as the after-burn. After intense exercise the body has to work hard to replenish energy stores and start the healing process. Exercise stresses the body, and in this case the stress is of a high degree, so the rest and sleep we have is of most importance to allow the body to adapt; making us stronger and fitter.

Core stability

Before we get started, let's define the meaning of core stability, as most of us know how to work it, or know of some exercises that will help to improve it, but what does it actually mean and just how important is it.

The meaning of the word core could be defined as 'the centre of a structure', for example; an apple core, or the core of the earth. When we use this word in relation to the body, we refer to the abdominal area, the area around the vertebral column between the ribs and the pelvis, known as the lumbar spine.

The term stability can be defined as supporting and stabilising a structure from unwanted movement, for example; the stability of a building is reliant on the supporting walls and pillars, another thought are the guide ropes for a tent to prevent it from collapsing, so when we discuss stability around the abdominal area of the body and spine, we are referring to the muscles and connective tissue that surround this area, and their ability to stabilise.

There are many muscles that we could include when talking about core stability, but we will list the main ones, these include:

Rectus abdominus (six pack)
Internal/external obliques (side abdominals)
Transverse abdominus (deep core muscle)
Erector spinae (spinal extensors)
Multifidus (spinal stabiliser)
Quadratus lumborum (spinal lateral stabiliser)

All these muscles work really hard during any exercise, particularly core stability exercises. Tranverse abdominus (the deepest of the abdominal muscles) will contract milliseconds before any other muscle contracts, this is a built in mechanism that acts to assist in the stabilisation and support of the spine, because with every move we make, all strength and power we produce comes from our core, and therefore is considered our centre of power.

There are many fancy core stability exercises out there that people do and encourage others to do, but the question you need to ask yourself is, "are these exercises really very functional?" Let's take for example the plank, probably the most common core stability known to man, in a face down (prone) position, either on your forearms or hands, you stabilise your whole body keeping it straight. So yes it will work your abdominals and core muscles, but how might this help you in any given situation? Ok, so it would be more beneficial to do it than to not do it, but is there another way in which we could work on core stability? Perhaps we need to be more dynamic when considering core stability exercises, because it doesn't have to be about keeping still, and more often than not we require core stability in a dynamic context rather than a static one, for example; when performing deadlifts and squats.

When prescribing and performing core stability exercises, whether static or dynamic, there are factors to affect the effectiveness of a particular exercise, and it is very important that we are aware of these. We should also ensure the client has been screened and cleared for exercise, and that the core stability exercises that we prescribe are appropriate to them and specific to their needs.

- ➢ Base of support. The more points of contact we have to the floor, the higher degree of stability we will have, as will the size of the point of contact. For example; sitting on a swiss ball with feet planted on the floor shoulder width apart will offer greater stability than if you were to lift one leg up, leaving you with the ball and one leg on the floor for support. Take both feet off the floor and you're likely to look like a circus balancing act as you shift forward and backwards and side to side to help keep your balance.
- ➢ Floor surface. The type of floor surface you perform your exercises on will make a huge difference. Imagine trying to balance on one leg on a thick exercise mat, compared to a

solid surface. This would put a lot more stress on the foot as the ankle worked hard to stabilise from unwanted movement. This can often be used to reduce stability and increase the effectiveness, for example; the use of a stability disc.
- Type of equipment. There are many types of equipment on the market that can be used, and are designed to be used for core stability. The type of equipment will affect the effectiveness of the exercise, for example; performing an abdominal curl on a swiss ball will prove to be more challenging to the core muscles than performing it on a BOSU solid side down; which is similar to a swiss ball, but more stable. Performing an abdominal curl on the floor will offer almost no instability.
- Fitness level. Fitness level and experience of the client is something to consider when prescribing core stability exercises. Many clients who may not have ever performed core stability exercises, or any exercise at all, will find the most basic of core exercises a challenge, whilst other more experienced clients can perform much more intense and unstable exercises.

Stretching

Stretching is simply taking two ends of a muscle as far about from each other as possible, and by doing this on a regular basis we can begin to see improvements in our flexibility and range of movement around a joint. Out of all the components of physical fitness, stretching must be the one that generally gets the least attention. The benefits of stretching definitely out-weigh the benefits of not stretching; including improved posture, reduced risk of strains and muscle tears, increased range of movement, and perhaps increased performance. The only disadvantage of stretching may be that it takes a little bit of time to perform, and as everybody these days are so time conscious, an extra ten minutes on the treadmill or a few more sets on the free-weights is favoured against boring stretching!

Static

Static stretching is the safest form of stretching and this type of stretch will suit everyone; it doesn't require much co-ordination and can be quite simple to perform. If you were to stretch the quadriceps statically, you would bring your heel to your bum by holding around the ankle, keep your knees in line and together, hold it there keeping it still while the muscle very gradually increased in length. This type of stretching is most common in gyms and where space may be limited. Static stretching can also be performed on the floor when appropriate, and this can help with relaxation.

Dynamic

Dynamic stretching is a very useful way to stretch, not commonly performed in a gym but much more common in a class environment or outside. One of the main advantages to this type of stretching is keeping warm. When you warm up before stretching, the heart rate is elevated and blood is pumped to the working muscles, but once you start stretching (statically), your body begins to cool down. When you stretch dynamically, you remain warm by way of the body moving during the dynamic stretches. A dynamic stretch still encourages a full range around the joint, but it is done with movement, for example; to stretch the quadriceps, all I need to do is shift my body weight from side to side and as I do so, raise each heel to my bum alternately by bending my knees and keeping my knees in line. There is no holding during dynamic stretching; the movement should allow you to smoothly move in and out of the stretch continuously. The only disadvantage this type of stretching may bring; is that due to its dynamic nature, there is an element of skill involved, usually co-ordination and balance, and because of this, people who are not accustomed to dynamic stretching may find they do not get such as an effective stretch.

Ballistic

Ballistic stretching is a very effective method of increasing flexibility, however it does come with higher risk of injury; this is because the stretch reflex (a safety mechanism to prevent muscles from over-stretching by contracting the lengthening muscle) cannot act quickly enough against this powerful and momentous lengthening of the muscle. It is characterised by bouncing or uncontrolled movements around a joint, for example, standing with your feet together and legs straight, leaning forward from your hips and using momentum to uncontrollably reach your feet or the floor in a bouncing type way. Perhaps if you have ever seen a Bruce Lee movie, you would have seen him preparing for a fight by swinging his leg high up in the air!

This type of stretching is very specific to sports as it prepares and lengthens the muscle by performing movements that usually mimic the sport. One thing to consider at this moment is that static stretching can actually reduce power output of the muscle, now as far as the average health related fitness client is concerned, this poses no issue, however, for the sports person, who may rely on a fraction more power to win the match or game; this is vital, but then for the elite athlete, the prize or the winning outweighs the risks involved, this is why you may have never seen a sports person doing static stretches before they perform, but never say never!

As fitness professionals of health related fitness, we have a duty of care towards our clients, and unnecessarily encouraging our clients to stretch this way may breach that rule. Ballistic stretching should not be performed by beginners to exercise and de-conditioned clients. Sports men and women in particular train very hard and their sport requires a range of ballistic actions which they will practice in training and during the game, match or heat, therefore, they have become accustomed to it and have reprogrammed the stretch reflex to deal with this degree of resistance and tension.

Myofascial release

Each muscle fibre, bundle of muscle fibres and whole muscle, is surrounded by a fascia or sheath, a very strong connective tissue which covers all muscles from head to toe in a continuous wrap. It is this fascia that causes the majority of tightness in muscles and is responsible for restrictive movement; therefore it is desirable to stretch this fascia in order to relieve stress and tension in the muscle. Stretching this fascia can also assist and help muscle growth, and it does this by allowing more room for the muscle to grow.

Myofascial release is a very effective method of stretching and relieving stress within a muscle, it is very similar to massage, and usually a foam roller will be used, but other equipment can be used in the same way, for example; a tennis or golf ball. Where stretching focuses on the whole muscle, myofascial release focuses on a single area, the intense pressure forced upon the muscle and connective tissue creates excessive tension which activates the golgi tendon organs (proprioceptor responsible for monitoring tension in the muscle), this triggers a higher state of relaxation; allowing the muscle and fascia to lengthen. This action, can also sooth out any knots in the muscle and tightness within the fascia, reducing excessive tension.

PNF (proprioceptive neuromuscular facilitation)

This method of stretching was used originally by physiotherapists to assist in recovery of stroke patients. It is a very effective way of stretching and developing range of movement around a joint if done correctly. In my experience I have seen many personal trainers assisting clients with this type of stretching, but unfortunately some of these trainers adopt a very inappropriate position with their client. It is difficult to judge whether the PNF stretch is being performed correctly and whether it is effective, but even if it is performed correctly, I have seen trainers straddle and lean over clients and for some this could be most intimidating, but my thought on this is that some trainers see it as a way of looking professional; I'm not so sure. Some clients may want to be treated like this, and maybe they are not bothered about personal space, however, when we deliver PNF stretching, whether we are assisting or not, we must respect our clients' personal space and remain professional.

CR (contract relax)

Initially the client is advised to take the muscle to its fullest range of movement, the trainer will then assist by holding the limb and resisting any movement as the client contracts the muscle to be stretched; this is usually done for about 10 seconds at approximately 50 percent of clients' ability. This action fires up the golgi tendon organs (propriocectors in the tendon) that detect the amount of tension within the muscle and work by inhibiting further force place against it (reciprocal inhibition), this allows the muscle to completely relax and allows a bigger range of movement to occur around the joint. After the 10 seconds, the client is told to relax and go further into the stretch, taking the joint to a new range of movement, and more often than not the trainer will usually assist at this stage, however, as the trainer, you must be aware of the clients range of movement and capability, thus not to force a muscle too much that it could result in injury; experience at doing this is key. The whole process could be done 3-4 times, as long as the client is comfortable and more importantly the muscle remain warm.

CRAC (contract relax antagonist contract)

This method is very similar to the CR method; the only difference here is, after the 10 second contraction, the antagonist (opposing muscle) contracts in order to help bring about a larger range of movement. So as an example; if you are lying on your back with on leg in the air stretching the hamstrings, the opposing muscles, hip flexors and rectus femoris are contracting, pulling the leg further into the stretch.

<u>When should we stretch?</u>

Ideally, we should stretch at the beginning of our workout after the warm up, this is usually called the prep stretch, and should only be performed once we are warm. Cold muscles do not respond well to stretching, so remember, we warm up to stretch, we don't stretch to warm up; as many people do.
Static, dynamic and ballistic stretching are most commonly performed at the start of a workout because they are quick to perform and usually mimic the movements in the main workout, whereas static stretching, PNF and myofascial release is recommended for the end of the workout.

The American College of Sports Medicine (ACSM) recommend the following guidelines for stretching.

Frequency – minimum of 2-3 times per week

Intensity – 2-3 reps per muscle group. Without inducing discomfort

Time – 15-60 seconds for static. 10-30 second assisted PNF

Type – static, dynamic or PNF (ballistic considered for sports)

Source: ACSM guidelines to fitness testing and exercise prescription, 8th edition (2010)

Session structure

Any exercise programme will always have three main elements to it, these are; warm up, main component and cool down. The purpose of each section is very different, and these guidelines should always apply whether it is sport specific or health related fitness.

The warm up component will consist of three sub-components; these are mobility, pulse raiser and prep stretch. During the warm up you are preparing the body for the main workout, the intensity may gradually increase to main workout level, but then that should indicate where the warm up has finished and the main workout has begin. Throughout the warm up, the joints around the body will also become warm, and the production and lubrication of synovial fluid will enable the joints to move smoothly whilst offering shock absorption from impact. As the body moves, the working muscles require more energy, and in this case, oxygen, so heart rate increases to supply the working muscles with more oxygen carried by the blood and pumped from the heart, and due to increased blood flow, the body, but more specifically the muscles get warm, this is known as the pulse raiser stage.

Warm muscles are much more receptive to stretching; and for reasons of health and safety, only at this stage of 'warm muscles' should stretching then take place. The main aim of the stretch in the warm up is to pre-lengthen the muscle, taking it through the range of movement expected in the main workout. Depending on the activity to follow; it may be wise in some cases to perform dynamic stretching in order keep the body warm and therefore reduce the cooling effect.
For some sports, the warm up may last for anything up to an hour, and the warm up may seem like a workout to some people, this is very specific to the individual and the sport. The warm up will also act as a skill rehearsal for the sport, preparing and warming up neuromuscular pathways. However, for general health related

fitness, it would be safe to say that fifteen minutes maximum is adequate for a warm up, focusing on the three elements and ensuring your client is physically prepared for the main workout.

Mental preparation is also a big reason for warming up, and if you are not in the correct frame of mind you do not perform as good as you could. Warming up prepares the mind and gets you over that 'I'm just not feeling it' stage, and usually once you get started you begin to feel glad you did.

During the main workout, cardiovascular or resistance training will take place, or even both, and this depends on the clients' goals and the exercise prescribed by the trainer. An appropriate higher level of intensity will be applied at this stage, gearing towards the clients goals. If the client is to focus on cardiovascular training, after the warm up, it will be necessary to re-warm the body in preparation for the higher intensity of the main workout, this is vital to ensure the cardiovascular system is operating effectively and the appropriate energy system (in this case aerobic energy system) is ready and working effectively.

As already mentioned; resistance training may form part of the main work out depending on the clients long and short term goals. If a cardiovascular and resistance training component is to be incorporated, then it may be usual to do the component that is most important first, for example; if aerobic fitness is the main goal, then the cardiovascular training would come first, however, it may be worth considering doing this component after the resistance if you want to pre fatigue the body and therefore making the aerobic component more challenging. This could also be said for the resistance training, and whilst some people may not agree with the idea, mixing up your workout in this way, along with other methods and training approaches will help to prevent the body from becoming stale and reaching a plateau.

Training the cardiovascular system only, keeps the structure of a workout relatively simple, and while you work hard in the main section, the cool down or pulse lowering that follows can act as the final part of exercise, leaving you with only the post workout stretches to do. If you only want to perform resistance training, there are a few considerations. It would be a good idea to perform one or two warm up sets at a light weight before performing the main set; to specifically warm up the joints and muscles associated with the exercise, and this can be particularly useful if you decide to completely skip the whole warm up component as mentioned earlier and want to get straight on with the exercise.

After your resistance workout you will need to stretch, but some muscles may have cooled down while you worked others, and therefore performing a re-warm would be very beneficial, this will help to flush out toxins that have accumulated in the muscles and will increase blood flow; warming the muscles up again, and therefore allowing them to be more susceptible to stretching.

The final part of any session that needs to take place is the cool down, and during this component you will most commonly include some pulse raising activities and some final stretches. As already mentioned, if only cardiovascular training is being performed, then the end of this component will act as your cool down and the body will remain warm enough to stretch, but if it doesn't, then a pulse raiser in the cool down is essential to re-warm the body in preparation for some final post workout stretches. The aerobic element will also help to clear toxins from the muscles and encourage faster recovery.

Stretching performed in the cool down will be aimed at maintaining and developing range of movement of muscles worked in the main workout, and ideally should be performed in a comfortable seated or lying position to help promote relaxation of the muscle being stretched.

See the example of how you might structure a workout for somebody who wants to incorporate aerobic and resistance training.

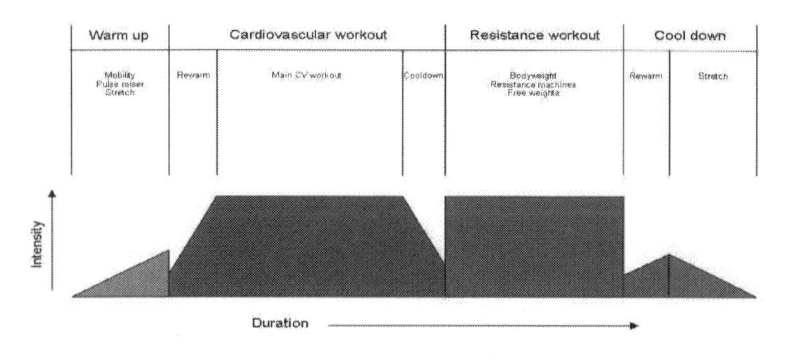

Progression

When it comes to progressing your clients programme, there are many ways in which to do it. There is no set formula for doing this and if one hundred trainers had to write a progressive programme for the same person you would end up with one hundred different programmes, they may have similar exercises throughout, but each one will have progression shown in a variety of ways based on different theories and personal experience. With the information you have taken on board from this book and your prior knowledge from formal training and experience, you should be equipped enough to make your own decision about how to plan and progress an exercise programme.

When progressing a programme or workout, it is worth knowing a selection of variables to help you gradually change and increase the intensity in order to ensure an adequate degree of overload is applied. Using the FITT principle (frequency, intensity, time and type) is a good place to start when; not only prescribing exercise, but also when you are progressing the programme. The FITT principle also acts as an overview of all variables.

The following variables will be appropriate for some forms of exercise but not for others, and therefore you will need to decide which is best suited.

Sessions per week
Sessions per day
Duration of session
Duration on equipment
Level
Incline
Resistance
Speed (kph, rpm and spm)
Distance
Repetitions
Rate (speed of movement)
Range of movement
% 1RM
Rest between sets
Type of equipment used

In order to increase our fitness, we must continue to progress our programme and more importantly the actual exercise. Sometimes it might be appropriate to maintain fitness; and in this case, keeping the training at a set level, in doing this, you continue to reap the benefits but fitness level remains the same. So the most common question asked is 'how often should I progress or change the programme?' Unfortunately the answer is not so simple, and there are many factors to affect the answer. One thing to consider is how long would it take you before you became bored of the same programme; let's say performing it three times a week? My personal thought on this would probably be about two weeks (six sessions) before I starting getting fed up with the very same programme.

With this said, it is no wonder why customers to a gym only follow their gym programme for a few weeks and then ignore it by doing their own thing which usually turns out to be something completely different, and the problem is because the gym instructor will write them a single programme; and this is no fault of the gym instructor. However, a good gym instructor will discuss with the customer how they can progress it and even encourage them to book in for a programme review, this is where progression is enforced and even a new programme designed.

So the question still stands, how often should we be progressing the programme? Well, unless the programme is periodised (long term goal broken up into different shorter term goals) then the programme should see a steady rate of linear progression, and this means that starting with the original programme, over a period of time, many of the variables come in and out of play, not to make one big change, but rather many small changes over an extended period of time.

By gradually changing and progressing the programme, it doesn't only keep the programme fresh, but also ensures that it is progressive. 4-6 weeks is a common time frame for programme change amongst trainers and exercisers, however, if this is the case then it is likely that the programme is either going to be periodised or just changed to add some variety, and variety should only be introduced for a reason and not just for variety!
As mentioned before, in a gym environment the use of one programme card is common, not to say that there isn't anyone who

uses multiple programme cards; because I have written plenty myself, but if a client is going to train three to four times per week, then using the same programme four times per week for six weeks is just ridiculous, apart from becoming very boring there is also the chance of overtraining if the same areas are worked in close concession. This is where the use of a split routine may help, and the idea of a split routine is to focus on different areas on different days, for example; a really common three day split routine may look something like this:

Monday - chest and triceps
Wednesday - back and biceps
Friday - legs and abs

Exercise is a form of stress on the body and too much of it can lead to long term health issues, and overtraining occurs when not enough rest is taken between days of exercise. The fact that most people ignore is that you do not get fitter as you train; you get fitter when you rest, this is the principle of adaptation, and these adaptations only take place as the body rests and recovers from exercise sessions. The body recognises all forms of stress as negative and so adapts in order to reduce the impact it causes next time, and this is the way in which we improve our fitness.

If the intensity in which you train is of that you are accustomed to and overload is not being applied, this is a level in which the body is used to and the stress placed upon it is minimal, this would explain why people at different fitness levels can continue to exercise for many consecutive days without overtraining, and why we can all do what we do day to day, particularly for some people with very active professions. With this said, even if we are not over stressing the body through exercise, many of us live life and work in the fast lane, and this is also a form of stress, so therefore we still need to take a break, visit the pit stop and have a rest day. It is recommended, even with a split routine that balances out all muscle groups and provides plenty of rest days for each; that you still take at least one day of complete rest.

The issue here is; that exercise can become very addictive, and sometimes people just want to train and train. The fact that we need rest to recover becomes non-existent to some of us and we feel so motivated to continue that we see having a day off will hinder our level of fitness and not enhance it, so therefore we just keep hitting the gym, unaware that our body's are reaching a level of stress where the first stages and side effects of overtraining occur. It is really important that these people are educated in understanding why we need to rest in between training sessions.

There may be many cases of people who you know that train day after day without rest and never get ill or injured, well the truth is, they are either not training hard enough or they will eventually. Every three steps of the ladder we climb, we must step back down one for recovery, it is crucial, and following this advice you will actually notice more physical and visual gains.

Evaluation

In order to be the best trainer you can be, it is vital that in some shape or form you reflect on your teaching and sessions taught in order to identify things that worked well and areas you can improve on. The truth is that we constantly reflect and evaluate on events that take place in our lives; whether it is wondering if you made the right decision buying those expensive shoes or repeating an argument over and over in your head and wondering if you could have handled it differently. So after you deliver a session with a client it would be worth evaluating to identify whether you could have done anything differently or better. The main reason we want to do this is to enhance the client experience, which will in turn hopefully keep them coming back for more. Doing this will also assist in your self-development, delivery and teaching of sessions. We have a few ways in which we can evaluate our sessions and teaching:

Feedback from the client

First hand feedback from the client is the best way to evaluate your session, however, it is client specific, meaning, what one client likes or doesn't like about your teaching and delivery is not going to be the same as another client. This is when you have to filter the feedback into two categories; the exercises, and your teaching. The use of open ended questions is vital when you gain feedback as most clients will keep their responses to a minimum, so be sure to gain lots of information from them.

Feedback from peers

Gaining feedback from your peers is a good way to evaluate your teaching, but obviously does require the time of the third party to observe you throughout a whole session. This may usually happen if you are to be observed or shadowed delivering your first session to a customer for a new employer, or as a practical assessment before you are employed, and many employers these days want to see you teach before they take you on. For an employer, safety and effectiveness from their gym staff is important, however, motivation and the way you speak with customers is at the top of their list and is one of the main reasons why customers will return.

Video footage

Trying to imagine how your session was for the client is a good form of evaluation, but video recording your session would allow you to see exactly how you acted and what you said to instruct and motivate. Just you watching yourself may help to identify areas that went well and some areas that need improving, but you may be guilty of being slight biased towards yourself and think how wonderful the session was, but if you were to observe it with a peer then you could discuss together how it went, then your opinion and evaluation would be much more constructive. If you are going to do any kind of video recording, you must ensure you have permission from the venue and consent from any person who may appear in the video, intentionally or unintentionally.

Chapter 8

Nutrition

As a personal trainer, many of your clients will want to seek nutritional advice from you to help them achieve their goals, so it is really important that you have a qualification before you start giving this advice. Most training providers will have a nutrition module bolted on to their personal trainer certificate, however, many may not, and unfortunately for the public, there are many trainers out there giving incorrect advice, believe me, I have heard it! Just because someone is a personal trainer with a level 3 qualification, it doesn't automatically mean they know anything about nutrition. For your own peace of mind, get yourself a nutrition certificate before giving advice to clients, the last thing you want is to end up in court with a lawsuit against you because you gave the wrong advice to someone.

So before you start giving nutritional advice, get yourself qualified with an appropriate qualification. As a personal trainer, your clients will expect you to know everything about nutrition (not that you should), but you should possess an exercise nutrition qualification, and most training providers will embed this qualification within a personal trainer course. If you are already qualified without nutrition, you can still attend a stand-alone nutrition module, and the following basic information is not adequate as training but only as a guide.

Macronutrients

These are what make up the bulk of our diet and are consumed in relatively large quantities, they consist of: carbohydrate, fat, protein and water. The figures, recommendations and suggestions that follow are general guidelines for the average person and should be varied on every individual in respect of their needs and physical activity levels.

Carbohydrates

These should constitute around 55-60% of our overall calories. The main role of carbohydrate is to supply the body with energy, and also to add fibre to our diet which will assist in the digestion process by creating bulk in our intestines, cleaning as it passes through and slowing down transit to help increase absorption of nutrients. Certain fibres can also help with improving cholesterol levels in the blood. Carbohydrate is categorised into two forms; complex and simple sugars.

Complex carbohydrates or sugars can be found in foods such as pasta, rice, potatoes, bread, fruit and vegetables and cereals. These types of carbohydrate contain fibre as well as other vitamins and minerals to ensure normal functioning of many bodily processes. Complex carbohydrates generally release their sugars into the blood slowly, keeping our energy levels fairly steady and keeping us feel fuller for longer, this is because of the fibre in the food we eat makes digestion harder, remaining in the stomach for longer, and also longer to pass through the gut.

We also get carbohydrates from our simple sugars, and these can be found in many foods, such as; sweets, fizzy drinks, cakes, biscuits and chocolate. As far as providing the body with carbohydrates, ATP production does not care where these carbohydrates (broken down into glucose) come from, however, if we consume simple sugars, these are termed as 'empty calories', and contain no nutrients, but they do contain many calories. Over consumption of simple sugars can lead to diabetes and obesity if consumed over a long period of time. These so called empty calories will very quickly and dramatically increase your blood sugar levels; demanding the release of insulin from the pancreas. Soon after consumption, blood sugar levels will drop low and the feeling of wanting more will dawn upon you again.

Protein

The role of protein is to build and repair bodily tissue, and is one of the most important aspects of training for some people. Protein plays a huge role in the body, such as; hormone, cell and cholesterol production, growth and repair of muscle tissue and used as an energy source. Protein can account for around twenty percent of total body weight and should make up approximately 10-15% of our dietary intake. We can and do use protein for energy, this is not desirable, but does happen during strength and endurance training whether we like it or not. For this reason, strength and endurance athletes are encouraged to take on more protein to allow for this offset, however, strength trainers do require more than endurance trainers; resulting in a requirement of 1.6-1.8 grams per kilogram of bodyweight for strength, compared to 1.2-1.4 grams per kilogram for endurance.

Fat

Fat should make up approximately 25-30% of our diet and plays a series of important roles to keep us healthy, for example; transmission of nerve impulses, insulation, absorption of certain vitamins and a fuel for aerobic energy production. The use of the word 'fat', however we use it, tends to be a negative thing, but without it, we wouldn't survive. The negativity around fat comes from the type of fat we consume that is considered bad for us, these are saturated and trans-fats. Saturated fat comes mostly from animal sources, but can be found in coconut and palm oil. Saturated fat is usually characterised as 'hard at room temperature', such as the fat found on red meat, lard, butter and cheese. We do not need this particular fat in our diet, and therefore it should only contribute to no more than 25% of overall fat consumed. However, there has been much research and documentation into the consumption of saturated fat, and with no hard evidence available to state it is really bad for you, many healthy people of a good weight swear on a diet high in this type of fat. The fat we should definitely stay away from is the trans-fats or hydrogenated fats; this type of fat has an unstable molecular structure; our body's do not recognise this man-made fat and is actually harmful to our health. If you eat processed foods, biscuits, cakes etc, you can be sure that you're getting your fair share. This fat is used highly in the food industry, as it prolongs shelf life and helps food to gel or stick together. Trans-fat is produced by taking unsaturated fat through the hydrogenation process, heating it up and cooling it down until it becomes the correct consistency. An example of this is the use of deep fat fryers for home frying. At the start, you fill it with clean and runny vegetable oil (unsaturated fat), but after a few uses it begins to solidify at room temperature. Pure unsaturated fats are the types of fat we should focus on and constituting for the majority of our fat intake. These unsaturated fats can be divided into two further categories, these are; monounsaturated and polyunsaturated fat. These types of fat should make up the majority of our fat intake, and these are considered to be healthy fats. You will find unsaturated fats in foods such as olives, seeds, avocados, oily fish and nuts. Essential fatty acids are found in polyunsaturated fat, and are more commonly known as omega 3 and omega 6, these play a vital role in health and well being, and must be consumed in our diet as our bodies cannot make it, however, omega 9 (not commonly known) is not termed an essential fatty acid, as our bodies can manufacture it.

Vitamins and minerals

Vitamins and minerals are classed as micronutrients, organic compounds that are found in a variety of foods in very small amounts; and these play specific roles within the body, helping it to function optimally. When we think about vitamins and minerals, you may visualise plastic bottles filled with tablets in almost any high street health food shop. These can prove to be very useful if you are deficient in a particular vitamin or mineral, and you need to supplement additionally, however, more often than not you will be recommended to get your intake of vitamins and minerals from fruit and vegetables and other 'real' foods.

We can divide vitamins into two categories, water soluble and fat soluble. Water soluble vitamins cannot be stored in the body so we need to consume a larger amount, and generally, an over consumption will leave the body in our urine. On the other hand, fat soluble vitamins are stored in the liver and fatty tissue, and are mainly found in fatty foods such as animal produce. Over consumption of fat soluble vitamins are stored for future use and an excessive store of these vitamins can be harmful.

There are many types of the B vitamin and they all have important roles to play, however, below you will find the main functions of them all.

Minerals are also divided into two categories, these are: macro elements (we require in greater amounts) and trace elements (we require in very small amounts).

The below table will help you to identify the different types of vitamins and minerals and give you a general overview of their function and best sources. Please note that this list of functions and sources are not exhaustive; but just a guide.

Vitamin	Function	Source
A (fat soluble)	Essential for good vision Strengthening immunity Antioxidant	Cheese, eggs, yogurt
B (water soluble)	Helps to release energy from food Healthy nerves and muscles	Pork, poultry, fish, potatoes and vegetables, peanuts, wheat, soya bean, eggs and meat
C (water soluble)	Supports the immune system Healthy cells and connective tissue Antioxidant	Fruit and vegetables, particularly oranges, strawberries, broccoli, red and green peppers and potatoes
D (fat soluble)	Healthy bones and teeth	Sunlight, fortified foods, oily fish and eggs
E (fat soluble)	Protection of cell membranes	Plant oils, nuts, seeds and cereals

	Antioxidant	
K (fat soluble)	Blood clotting	Green leafy vegetables, vegetables and cereals

Mineral	Function	Source
Calcium	Building strong bones and teeth Muscle contraction	Nuts, soya drinks, milk, cheese and green leafy vegetables
Sodium	Body fluid balance	Small amount found in all food Processed food and ready meals
Magnesium	Muscle and nerve impulse, blood glucose control	Green leafy vegetables, fish, meat, dairy foods and nuts
Potassium	Body fluid balance	Bananas, nuts and seeds, milk, fish and pulses
Zinc (trace)	Healthy immune system Helps make new cells and membranes	Meat, milk and dairy, shellfish and bread
Selenium (trace)	Immune system function Antioxidant	Nuts, fish and eggs

Copper (trace)	Red and white blood cell production Helps to form haemoglobin	Nuts and shellfish
Chromium (trace)	Affects the amount of energy we get from food	Wholegrains, spices, broccoli and potatoes

Phytonutrients

Phytonutrients are natural compounds found in fruit, vegetables, grains and legumes that play a vital role in promoting good health. There are hundreds of phytonutrients, and these are often referred to as phytochemicals, and many of these have antioxidant properties, neutralising free radicals in the body and preventing cell damage, some phytonutrients have also been shown to reduce the risk of heart disease. Some examples of food that are rich in phytonutrients include: bright and colourful fruit and vegetables, dark green leafy vegetables, wholegrain foods, nuts, seeds, soya bean and legumes.

Food fortification

'Fortified with vitamins and minerals is a term most of us hear about and read on food labels, especially cereal box's; but what it actually means is what many of us are not so sure about. Food fortification or enrichment is defined by the World Health Organisation (WHO) as 'The practice of deliberately increasing the content of an essential micronutrient, i.e. vitamins and minerals (including trace elements) in a food irrespective of whether the nutrients were originally in the food before processing or not, so as to improve the nutritional quality of the food supply and to provide a public health benefit with minimal risk to health'.
Food fortification was identified by the World Health Organisation (WHO) and Food and Agricultural Organisation of the United

Nations (FAO) as a means of reducing deficiencies of essential nutrients on a global level. The most common fortified foods are: cereals, milk and milk products, fats and oils, infant formulas and hot and cold beverages.

Creatine

Creatine is an energy compound made by the body and stored in the muscle that we use as a fuel for the phospho-creatine energy system. Some weight trainers supplement it in their diet to boost their stores in preparation for a hard weight training session, giving them 'extra' energy to perform better for longer, however it can also be found in meat that we consume, so taking a supplement is not essential. A break from creatine supplementation is advised, so the body knows it still has to produce it, as continuous use may fool the body into thinking it doesn't need to. The phospho-creatine energy system is responsible for short, fast, powerful, explosive and high intensity activities, for example; weight training (low reps), 100m sprint and throwing and jumping, it can only work for very short periods of time and takes a considerable amount of time to replenish depleted stores, unlike glycogen. Be aware that creatine supplementation does not work for everyone and can cause water retention, and if you decide to try it, ensure you read the guidelines to taking it very carefully.

Glycaemic Index (GI)

The glycaemic index is a scale of 1-100, and is based on what effect a carbohydrate based food has on blood sugar levels. A slow absorbing food will have a low GI rating, and a fast absorbing food will have a high GI rating. Slow releasing foods are important for a steady release of sugar into the blood, especially if you have diabetes. Glucose is used as the reference food and has a GI rating of 100, all other foods are compared to this. This scale was devised to assist diabetics in determining the best type of food to consume. There are many factors that will affect the GI rating of a food, these include: how the food is cooked, i.e. frying, boiling and baking, the ripeness of particular fruit and vegetables, whether a food is wholegrain, wholemeal or refined, fat lowers the GI of a food, protein lowers the GI of a food, dairy products are high in fat due to their high protein and fat content.

A low GI diet is not generally recommended; it may be unbalanced and high in fat, instead, focus on a balanced diet that is low in fat and sugar, and contains plenty of varied fruit and vegetables.

Water and hydration

Water makes up approximately 60% of our body weight; it flows through our blood carrying nutrients and oxygen around the body and into cells. We constantly lose water through breathing, sweating, urinating and bowel movement. We can expect to lose between 1-2 litres of water per day so it is really important for us to constantly replenish it.

Water is responsible for temperature regulation, flushing out waste products and cushioning joints and soft tissue. Water also plays a big part, and is vital for the process of digestion. A major side effect of dehydration is constipation, as the faeces dry up and can no longer pass through the large intestine; this is because the large intestine is the final site in the digestive system where water is extracted before secretion.

We can survive up to 3 weeks without food, but only 3 days without water before we perish, and the slightest amount of dehydration (3%) can have massive negative effects on our performance and concentration.

Water is found in many foods, however, we must get the majority from drinking it; it doesn't have to be plain water to remain hydrated, but be aware that many drinks contain caffeine, for example tea, coffee and many fizzy drinks, these will encourage the body to lose water, and could effectively have the opposite desirable effect.

Water intoxication

Consuming large amounts of water over a relatively short period of time can be potentially fatal as you flush out essential electrolytes.

Hyponatremia is the name given to this condition and translated is Latin for insufficient salt in the blood.

When we consume vast quantities of water, the liver cannot filter it fast enough, and therefore water enters the cells, and as these cells take on water they swell, and in areas of the body where there is no room for this, such as brain cells, leading to brain swelling, which manifests as seizures, coma, respiratory arrest and death. You may have heard of many cases of this condition from long distance runners who failed to appropriately rehydrate; it is also common for clubbers taking MDMA (ecstasy) to develop hyponatremia after trying to rehydrate following hours of dancing and sweating. Symptoms of water intoxication include headache, fatigue, nausea, vomiting, frequent urination and mental disorientation.

Approximately one sixth of marathon runners will experience dilution of the blood, or hyponatremia by drinking too much water. (New England Journal of Medicine, 2005)

Sports drinks

During continuous moderate to vigorous exercise the body dehydrates, losing water and essential electrolytes such as sodium and potassium through sweat, these electrolytes are needed by cells to carry electrical nerve impulses to other cells, and it is extremely important that these are all replaced during and after exercise, to avoid post workout fatigue.

You can go into any convenience store or supermarket and you will no doubt be able to purchase a sports/energy drink of some kind, but do you really know enough about them in order to make an educated guess as to which one you should have? And let's be honest, there are so many to choose from, that you would be forgiven for making the wrong decision. Unfortunately, many people are drinking these types of drinks because they simply like them, and this is great news for the companies who make and sell them, but actually, not so great for the consumer. It's understandable that these sport and energy drinks taste nice, but the reason is because they have lots of sugar (energy) and many other ingredients in them, and this means calories, and too many calories mean weight gain!

Energy drinks

These types of beverage contain stimulant drugs such as caffeine; this drug stimulates the body and the mind. Some energy drinks contain up to 120mg of caffeine (more than three times the amount of cola), they also contain sugar, herbal extracts and amino acids; however, different brands will have varying ingredients and amounts. Taurine is a well-known ingredient in energy drinks and is a common amino acid, taurine supports neurological development and also helps control water and mineral salts in the blood. Some studies suggest that taurine improves sports performance, so perhaps this is why it is added to energy drinks.

Sports drinks

Isotonic sports drinks contain the same concentrations of sugar and salt as the blood, therefore providing hydration and a boost of carbohydrate for energy, this is most athletes favoured sports drink and is especially useful for middle to long distance runners.
Hypertonic sports drinks contain higher concentration levels of sugar and salt compared to blood, this helps to deliver a higher amount of carbohydrate; however, because of the increase in carbohydrate, the fluid is not absorbed, so it is advised to consume water alongside it. This type of drink would be ideal for someone taking part in a short duration, high intensity exercise, such as gymnastics
Hypotonic sports drinks contain a lower concentration of sugar and salt compared to blood, and because of this the fluid can be more easily absorbed; assisting in hydration, and the small amount of sugar will provide the body with a little energy, this would be ideal for a 60 minute gym session, where rehydration usually outweighs the need for additional energy.

Salt

Salt or sodium is an essential nutrient within our diet; it regulates water balance and is essential for correct nerve and muscle function. The worrying factor is that most people consume too much, this is due to it being very present in manufactured and processed foods, this helps to preserve it and also to give it a nice taste. Salt is also added during cooking and on the table, and most people will add it before even tasting the food, therefore this has become a habit for most people.

Over consumption of salt is not desirable, because as we consume excessive amounts of salt, it causes the blood to become thicker; and to counteract this, the body draws in more fluid, and in turn causes blood pressure to increase. Recommended daily amounts of salt, is 6mgs, and that is approximately a teaspoon measure.

Encourage your clients to check and monitor the amount of salt they are consuming by following these guidelines:

- Check food labels for salt content
- Reduce amount used in cooking
- Eat more natural/organic food
- Opt for low salt options
- Taste before adding at the table

Alcohol

Alcohol is a non-essential nutrient that has no positive effects on our health and we can live without; however it does have some positive effects, these include; improving mood and increasing confidence.

Moderate amounts of alcohol have been shown to have no negative effects on health, but consuming large amounts are linked to liver damage and increased weight. Alcohol contains 7 calories per gram with no nutritional value; add your favourite mixer and you have a cocktail for a potentially high calorific drink.

Alcohol is a diuretic, which means it will encourage your body to lose water, and ultimately dehydrate you. Excessive alcohol consumption will leave you very dehydrated and also low on essential electrolytes, resulting in headaches and lethargy, consuming food whilst you are drinking will help to keep sugar and salt levels up and could reduce the hangover effect. Drinking water as well as your favourite alcohol will reduce the dehydration effect, if this proves to be inconvenient: then ensure you drink a pint of water before retiring to bed. Good luck with not having to get up in the night to wee!

Government guidelines for safe alcohol consumption (the amount you can safely drink without affecting your health) are 14-21 units per week (2-3 units per day) for females, and 21-28 units per week (3-4 units per day) for males. Without looking at the alcohol content and checking how many units you are consuming every time you go out; get an idea of how many units there are in your favourite beverage. The alcohol strength and size of drink will determine the amount of units it equates to.

BMR (basal metabolic rate)

Your basal metabolic rate or BMR relates to the amount of calories your body requires, in order to function at rest, this is also known as your metabolism. An individuals' BMR will depend on a few factors, these include; amount of muscle mass, age, height, gender, and the amount of exercise they participate in; stress and illness will also increase your metabolic rate.

A very simple method of calculating BMR, that used to be used, was; 25 x bodyweight in Kgs = BMR. You would then multiply this figure by 1.2 if you are sedentary, 1.5 if you are active and 1.75 if you were very active. As you can imagine, this is a very general way of calculating BMR and does not take individual factors into the equation. Below is a much more accurate method of calculating BMR which does take peoples weight, height and age into consideration.

BMR formula

Women
BMR = 655 + (9.6 x weight in kilos) + (1.8 x height in cm) - (4.7 x age in years)

Men
BMR = 66 + (13.7 x weight in kilos) + (5 x height in cm) - (6.8 x age in years)

Harris Benedict Equation

Using the Harris Benedict Equation allows you to apply the correct amount of activity that a person does, and this will tell us approximately how many calories they should be consuming on a daily basis.

Once you have calculated your BMR, multiply it by the following:

Sedentary (little or no exercise) BMR x 1.2
Lightly active (light exercise/sport 1-3 days per week) BMR x 1.375
Moderately active (moderate exercise/sport 3-5 days per week) BMR x 1.55
Very active (hard exercise/sport 6-7 days per week) BMR x 1.725
Extra active (very hard exercise/sport & physical job or 2x training) BMR x 1.9

Example:
Total daily calories for a moderately active individual to maintain current weight
BMR (1,700kcals) x 1.55 = 2,635kcals

The above example will give you an approximation of calories needed in order to maintain weight. Once this has been identified, you can then calculate how many calories needed to increase and reduce weight.

When calculating BMR and applying the Harris Benedict Equation, it is worth noting that these figures are accurate for lean bodyweight, and a leaner body requires more calories compared to a less lean (more fat) body, therefore, using this formula for a particularly muscular person will give you an underestimated number of calories, and for a less lean (fatter) person, you will have overestimated the amount of calories required.

Excess Post-exercise Oxygen Consumption (EPOC)

EPOC refers to the amount of calories burnt post exercise, and is more commonly known as the 'after burn effect'. After exercise, metabolism remains raised above normal levels whilst the body recovers from exercise, this can often be felt for several hours if the exercise intensity is high enough. It is thought that the reason this occurs is because the body is working hard to replenish creatine and glycogen stores and also beginning the process of adaptation, all these processes take energy, and in this case the energy source that is used is fat, if the exercise intensity is high enough, then a considerate amount of fat calories will be used long after exercise has ceased. Great news for when you are sitting relaxing watching your favourite television programme!

A study was conducted by Bahr and Sejersted (1992), where three groups of cyclists all cycled for 80 minutes but at different intensities to establish the relationship between exercise intensity and EPOC effect.

Exercise intensity	Approximate HR	Duration of EPOC
Light (29% VO2 max)	45%	0.3 hours
Moderate (50% VO2 max)	65%	3.3 hours
Vigorous (75% VO2 max)	80%	10.5 hours

Source: Bahr and Sejersted (1992)

This may answer the question that many clients ask regarding how hard they should be working, or at which level. The answer is simple, work as hard as you can for the given amount of time you have, and the harder you work during exercise, the more calories you burn during and after exercise.

Fat burning during aerobic exercise

If you are familiar with exercise and have done some research, spoken to someone in the gym, or seen some information on a CV machine, you will be familiar with the fact that low intensity exercise burns the most amount of fat. For that reason, it is very common to see many people, particularly in a gym, working at a low level of intensity, and when you ask them what they are trying to achieve, they will tell you that they are on a fat loss programme to lose weight, and they have been told that they need to work at low intensity in order to do this. Ok, so this is true, working at low intensities of exercise, usually around 55-70% max HR will actually burn the most fat, however, low intensity exercise will burn the largest 'percentage' of calories from fat, but not necessarily a large amount overall, for example; if an exercise used 50% of its calories from fat but only used 15 calories overall, that ends up not sounding like such a great deal!

For a beginner, working at a low level of intensity is recommended, usually 55-70% MHR, but as an individual gets fitter, it is no longer appropriate for them to work at such a low intensity, and therefore the intensity needs to be increased, if it isn't, then a plateau will be reached and no further cardiovascular benefits will be gained, not to mention the fat loss benefits. People will still insist on working at this low level as it apparently burns more fat.
Take a look at the diagram on the next page.

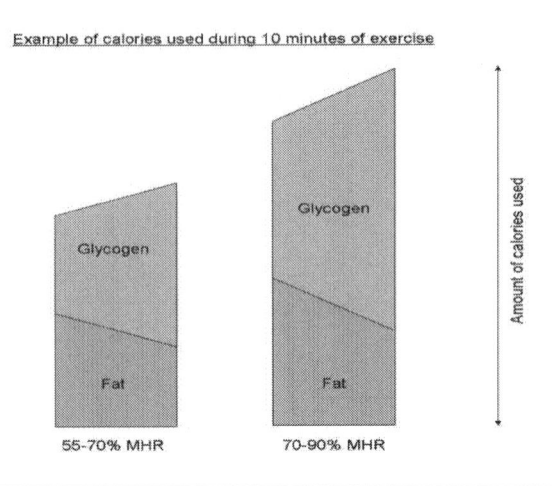

Example of calories used during 10 minutes of exercise

55-70% MHR	70-90% MHR
Glycogen / Fat	Glycogen / Fat

Amount of calories used

As you can see from the diagram above, during low intensity exercise; the percentage of calories from fat are much higher than that of high intensity exercise. However, during higher intensity exercise, you are using a much larger amount of calories, and even though the percentage of fat calories is lower, this means you will end up utilising more fat calories overall.

Beginners to exercise will initially use a much higher percentage of calories from glycogen (glucose stored in the muscle), and they do not have the ability to effectively utilise fat as a fuel. And therefore it is more appropriate to start a beginner at a lower level of intensity, whether their goal is fat loss or not. If intensity levels are too high, then a high percentage of glycogen calories are used and the exerciser will experience fatigue after a short duration of exercise. Fat cannot be utilised as a fuel for aerobic exercise when glucose is not present, so it is important that we educate clients regarding this, as the belief of not eating will encourage the body to use up more body fat still exists.

Digestion

Digestion is the mechanical and chemical process of passing food through the digestive system; absorbing water and nutrients from it.

This process starts at the mouth as we chew the food in order to break it into smaller pieces; making later digestion easier, this is called mastication, and during this time the salivary glands secrete saliva which contains an enzyme called amylase, this is responsible for the first process of chemical digestion of carbohydrates. After chewing approximately twenty times (recommended), we produce a ball of food ready to swallow, this is called a bolus. As we swallow the bolus, it passes down the oesophagus with the help of muscular contractions called peristalsis until it meets the door of the stomach, this is actually a valve that opens and closes in response to food, however, some people have a problem with their valve not closing, which causes reflux, acid from the stomach escaping up through the food pipe and giving a burning sensation; known as heart burn.

Once the ball of food has entered the stomach it is greeted by a cocktail of digestive enzymes, such as; pepsin to digest protein, bile and lipase to break down and digest fat, and also hydrochloric acid. The stomach mixes the food and chemicals together to produce chyme; an acidic and liquid substance.

After spending a period of time in the stomach, the half digested food then enters the small intestine where further digestion takes place. As food passes along the small intestine, the body begins to absorb the nutrients from the food, and the slower the movement of food through this part of the intestine; the higher the absorption rate. This is where the need for fibre comes in, as it slows down the transit speed of food by adding bulk and cleaning the digestive tract along the way, making it more efficient at absorbing nutrients.

As the digested food leaves the small intestine it enters the large intestine (or colon), this is where water and sodium is finally absorbed. Any undigested food and waste is packed together to form faeces, and when this reaches the rectum (the final section of the digestive tract) we feel the urge to visit the toilet and finally remove it via the anus.

Chapter 9

Bad habits in the gym

The purpose of this section is to make you aware of bad habits that people pick up and also certain behaviours you will experience from working in a gym. I have no doubt whatsoever that you will experience some if not all of these habits. You may even decide to use some of these for creating your own gym rules. Some of the following are actions that may distract and upset other users, whilst others are health and safety issues that should be addressed before people are allowed in the gym.

Dropping weights

This is an issue that every single gym faces, it is one of the most common and also one of the most annoying habits that a number of people have whilst using free weights. The funny thing is that I do understand why people do it sometimes, but at the same time cannot understand why people do it, let me explain.
If you are a regular gym user (especially in the free weights area) you'll know exactly what I'm talking about, and you may even be one of these people. The regular weight dropper will usually perform an exercise on a bench, and rather than lowering it down to the ground slowly, they drop them from a height, sending it crashing to the floor. Let's look at this issue from an athletes' point of view; for example a power lifter or even the worlds' strongest man competition; a power lifter will attempt one lift from the floor using massive amounts of strength, power and momentum in order to shift a ridiculously heavy weight, and what do they do once they have lifted it? Yes you're right, they just drop it down to the floor, why? Because they couldn't possibly put this weight down in a safe way! The sport is about being able to lift a weight and not lowering it, so therefore why would they possibly risk putting it down slowly, they just let go and walk away. The Olympic bars used by these athletes are reinforced, as are the platforms and floors this sport is performed

on, they are built to take massive amounts of impact. I think you may be starting to realise where I am going with this?

The same applies with the worlds' strongest man competition, exactly the same thing, these monsters of strength throw their weights around in order to complete a task in the quickest time or as many repetitions in the given time, these athletes aren't judged on how they lower their weights and they certainly don't concern themselves with it either.

Ok, so back to the gym environment, and what I think we should consider first is the theory of eccentric training. An eccentric muscle contraction is when a muscle is tense and lengthening at the same time, you can perform an eccentric muscular contraction by lowering a weight down towards the floor, take for example a bicep curl (a bicep curl is always the easiest exercise to use), the eccentric phase is lowering the weight and your arms are extending after you have lifted it, try it now, pick something up and slowly lower it, see how your bicep muscle contracts but actually lengthens at the same time, there you go, an eccentric contraction. These types of contractions are actually easier to perform than the concentric type using the same weight, concentric contractions are the opposite and the muscle shortens as it contracts. Research has shown that we are approximately 40% stronger during the eccentric phase, meaning that lowering a weight is actually easier than lifting it. Many gyms have signs up on the walls and mirrors asking people not to drop the weights on the floor, but the best one I have seen is the one that identifies by not dropping weights and putting them away will actually make you stronger, how right they are!

The other thing to consider is damage to the floor and free weights, whilst some gyms have installed power lifting platforms in their free weights area, many gyms do not have this luxury, and when weights are continuously dropped from a height to the floor, they will inevitably get damaged. Gym owners do what they can to cushion and reinforce free weight room floors, but if continuous abuse from customers dropping weights is always going to happen, then no doubt something is going to break.

Bad attitudes

If you didn't know already, during resistance training (and endurance training), the male hormone testosterone is released into the blood, and in the gym environment this is a positive thing. The sensation and effects of testosterone will make you feel more confident and sometimes aggressive, but also give you a boost in strength.

Testosterone is a vital hormone produced in the testes of males to allow growth and masculinity. Some people have naturally low testosterone levels, but fear not because exercise does increase testosterone levels which may help towards maintaining long term levels.

It is the short term effects that we are most concerned with here, and during intense resistance training some people can appear totally unapproachable, look like they're going to smash their fist through the wall, or generally looking really angry and upset. This is ok as long as they understand why they are experiencing this heightened aggressiveness and can control it, not let other people feel intimidated by them and not to strut around the gym like they are invincible with their chest purposely lifted and shoulders swaying forward and back.

This, perhaps unintentional attitude and aggression can have a massive impact on others users within a gym; and whilst it may help others around them to lift more and perform more repetitions in a spit and sawdust gym, in a more common chain or council run gym, many people will find this behaviour intimidating, which may discourage them from using the free-weight area.

Moaning and groaning

Now before we get started on this one let me remind or educate you on the valsalva effect. The valsalva effect is a phenomenon that relates to the holding of breath during exercise. Some people do it on purpose to increase intra-abdominal pressure, whilst some people do it subconsciously. When it is done involuntarily we need to encourage people to maintain their breathing as this can cause a short term rise in blood pressure. We know that blood pressure rises in correspondence to exercise intensity, so avoiding any further short term increases in blood pressure seems desirable. If you are at all wondering what the implications of high blood pressure are, then I suggest you stop reading and go look it up right now!

So back to the issue in hand; moaning and groaning. If you have ever set foot in a gym this has to be one of the first things you are most likely to come across, or hear! So why do people do it? Well let me tell you, there is likely to be a number of reasons why people do it. The first reason is related to the valsalva effect as mentioned above, and because people will hold their breath to help achieve this intra-abdominal pressure sometimes the amount of force produced during a lift is so high that they find ourselves breathing out slowly but forcefully, this of course isn't the problem, the problem lies with how verbal someone will be as they do this. You may be lucky enough to be working out next to someone who manages to breath out quietly as they attempt their last 5 or 6 reps, or you may be unlucky enough to find yourself working out in the same gym to the person who has no awareness or consideration for other users of the gym and just yell out like a grizzly bear for every repetition. This can be very off-putting, intimidating and totally unacceptable in the gym environment.

During my time as a gym instructor I witnessed a couple of middle aged males who would come into the gym and make an excessive amount of noise whilst lifting weights, and what made this particular situation even worse was the fact that the gym itself was very small and therefore 'everyone' in the gym could hear them. But as mentioned earlier, they had absolutely no respect for others, eventually they had to be told, and although the need to discuss this matter with the guilty party was completely justified, they didn't take it too kindly and decided to cancel their membership in response, a very childish act but at least the rest of the members didn't have to listen to them anymore, nor me for that matter. Obviously you are better off losing 2 members than risking losing more and upsetting others along the way.

Working in a top London gym a good few years later I happen to experience the moaning and groaning of one lone male in the free weights room, luckily it wasn't my duty to approach the gentleman and have words, but the sound he used to make was very disturbing indeed, it wasn't particularly loud, but the only way I can really describe it was like he was making love to a beautiful women and groaning in ecstasy on every out breath!

Use of phones

Do you come to the gym to work out? Or do you come to the gym to play about with your phone, make or take telephone calls and take pictures of yourself working out? If you are going to work out then why take your phone?!

Sometimes we are expecting an urgent phone call and desperately need to keep our phones close by; fair enough, me too. If we happen to be in the gym then so be it, carry your phone around with you, but there is no need to constantly keep using your phone unnecessarily for the whole duration of your training session.
I have a belief that if you are serious about your training and you go to the gym to work on your fitness; then leave your phone in the locker, in your car or at home, it is a major distraction, not only for the owner but also for other people who are trying to get on with their work out and have to constantly listen to the sound of your message alert or ring tone.
Another issue with the use of phones in the gym is when people (usually young males) start taking pictures of themselves in the mirror; and I bet if you could see their Facebook home page one of those ridiculously vain pictures would be there. See next subject below.

Posing

What is the reason for people going to the gym? Hopefully you're already thinking of a similar answer to mine, which is to get fit, improve fitness, muscular strength, muscular endurance, cardiovascular fitness and improve sports performance? Whatever the reason, I'm happy people are attending the gym and getting themselves fitter. But why do people insist on posing and treating the gym like a modeling show? Now I'm guilty, and I'm sure nearly every other male is slightly guilty of having a sneaky look at themselves after a set of muscle pumping reps, of course we have, and as we exercise our muscles fill with blood, making them look bigger than normal, this is what I believe some people call 'pumped', and when we're pumped our muscles fill with extra blood to provide oxygen and nutrients to the working muscle, brilliant, but this only lasts for a limited period of time; but when it does occur it can certainly make us look bigger, just like we've achieved a massive episode of hypertrophy. This can be particularly helpful on a Friday night before we go out wearing a tight t-shirt with our 'guns' on show, in hope of a member of the opposite sex being unbelievably attracted to us; or maybe not!

If people want to pose then that's fine I really don't mind, but please don't do it in the gym, it is so off-putting and you run the risk of just looking like an idiot. This does only seem to happen when there are mirrors, and if there are no mirrors then the posing seems to be less.
The worst behaviour has to be the lifting of t-shirts in front of the mirror, and even worse taking a picture at the same time. It does make you wonder about the question I asked at the start though doesn't it?

Weights belts

We spoke earlier about the valsalva effect and the reason why this occurs. If you skipped that bit may I suggest that you go back and read it, unless of course you know exactly what it is, and you're not interested in my opinion.

The use of weights belts is very common and very beneficial for experienced body builders and weight lifters alike, these athletes push themselves to their limit in order to train and compete at the highest levels, giving them maximum stability around the mid-section of the body; 'the weakest link' as I like to call it.

One consequence of lack of support during this type of training at a high intensity can be a hernia, usually this will be in the form of an inguinal hernia; this is an area of the lower abdomen between the ilium and the pubic bone, the site of the inguinal ligament.

The problem for me lies on seeing the average exerciser using them. Now, let us not assume here that every person who wears a weights belt is a general exerciser that doesn't actually need it as we know assuming is the worst thing anyone can do, but so too often I see people wearing weights belts during regular exercise, maybe there is a very valid and justifiable excuse for this, perhaps they have been advised by a physiotherapist or doctor, or maybe they saw it on the internet and thought how good they may look wearing it in the gym, make them look the part, but why should they need to be using one?

For the general exerciser, a whole body approach to training should be used, and that includes core stability; whether you do it as a separate component or focus on it during every exercise you do. The fact is, that if you engage and focus on your core muscles in a way mentioned above, then you should have obtained a good degree of core strength, stabilising the lumbar spine and therefore reducing the need for a weights belt in the first place.

Inappropriate use of equipment

Resistance machines and other exercise equipment is made for a specific purpose, and this purpose is, 'to be used appropriately and the purpose it was designed for'.

At the time of writing this section of the book, I experienced an exerciser performing an exercise that could do so much damage and cause massive personal injury. The exercise that I experienced was a leg press on the smith machine, right now you may have no idea what I am talking about, if so, don't worry I will explain. The smith machine is a plate loaded resistance machine, this means you can load it up with multiple free weight plates; this makes it a fixed resistance machine with free-weight properties. The smith machine could usually be described as a cage, comprising of two sides in which an Olympic bar glides up and down in a vertical plane. This machine is usually used for bench press and many other effective exercises.

What I think is unacceptable and completely crazy to do (and I hope you'll agree) is a leg press on this machine, lying on the floor with the bar situated above the hips and with the feet pushing the bar, taking the legs into extension as the bar raises up. The smith machine has a safety feature where you can limit the bar from coming down too far, this is really important for client safety, however, during the use of this machine, and in this case an exercise that this machine isn't designed for, the use of this safety feature wasn't present. As an instructor you would only look and weep at this exercise and its safety implications.

As an instructor it is your role to check and reinforce correct use of equipment; for the health and safety of the user, and also for the longevity of the equipment.

Summary and close

I hope that you enjoyed reading this book; or parts of it, and found some of the content interesting and informative, and more importantly learnt something from it. If you read it for your own benefit and as an interest to you, then I hope it has inspired you to consider entering the fitness industry.

To the date of this book being published, I have been involved in the fitness industry for nearly fifteen years; it has been a journey to say the least as I have seen and personally experienced many changes. One of the things I like most about this industry is that it has so much to offer with so many different routes to take, I guess many occupations do for that matter, but how many do you know of that the majority of people like to do in their spare time? So on that note, this industry really is about doing something that you actually enjoy.
There may be a particular area or specialism within fitness that you are passionate about, if so, find out more about it; what it takes to get qualified and what you can then do with that qualification. Continue to develop your knowledge by reading lots of books, these do not necessarily have to be about fitness, but certainly related to it in some way. I found a passionate interest in psychology, and particularly in why people act in ways in which they do, this definitely helped me to break down communication and physical barriers with clients, and of course to try and understand them.
Good luck to you, wherever you go from here.
Please like my 'A Complete Guide to Personal Training' Facebook page and leave your comments. Many thanks.

Justin Bailly
Author

References:

http://www.exerciseregister.org

http://www.nhs.uk

http://www.diabetes.co.uk

http://www.weightlossresources.co.uk

http://www.mayoclinic.org

The Complete Guide to Sports Nutrition, 4th Edition, Anita Bean

The Optimum Nutrition Bible, Patrick Holford

Advanced Fitness Assessment and Exercise Prescription, 4th Edition, Vivian H. Heyward

Index

A
Advertising 22
Alcohol 148
Anaemia 76
Anorexia
Anthropometrics 60
Arthritis 74
Asthma 77

B
Ballistic stretching 125
Barriers 103
Basic set training 107
Berger 115
Blood pressure 62
Body mass index 59
Basal metabolic rate 149
Body composition 64
Body language 42
Borg scale 88

C
Calories 91
Cancellation policy 33
Carbohydrates 138
Cardiovascular fitness 51, 55
Circuit training 107
CHD 73
Cheat system 116
Children 96
Code of ethics 13
Communication 41
Competition 27
Components of fitness 50
Consultation 38
Continuing professional development 14
Continuous training 118

Cooper test 56
Core stability 122
Creatine 144
Curriculum vitae 15

D
Delayed onset muscle soreness 84
Delorme & Watkins 113
Diabetes 72
Digestion 153
Disability 98
Dose response 82
Drop sets 111
Dynamic stretching 125

E
Excess post-exercise oxygen consumption 151
Equipment 38
Evaluation 135

F
Fartlek training 120
Fat 139
Feedback 135
First aid 15
Fitness assessment 48, 55
Fitness instructing 8
Fitness principles 79
Flexibility 53, 57
Food fortification 143

G
Giant sets 109
Glycaemic index 144

H
Health assessment 59
Heart rate 64, 85

Heart rate zones 87
High intensity training 120
HMRC 27

I
Ice bath 85
Income tax 28
Informed consent 70
Interval training 119

K
Kinetic chain 80
Kyphosis 69

L
Listening skills 44
Lordosis 68

M
Macronutrients 137
Marketing 20
Metabolic equivalent of task 91
Minerals 140,142
Monitoring 85
Motor skills 53
Muscular endurance 52, 57, 106
Muscular strength 52, 57, 106
Myofascial release 126

N
National insurance 28
Negatives 112
Nutrition 137

O
Onset blood lactate accumulation 88
Obesity 73
Overload 79

Overtraining 79, 83
Older adult 95

P
Personal trainer 8
Phytonutrients 143
Plateau 8
Plyometrics 116
PNF 127
Post exhaust 110
Posture analysis 48, 67
Power training 117
Pre exhaust 110
Pregnancy 97
Pricing 32
Progression 132
Promoting yourself 26
Protein 138
Pyramid training 109

Q
Qualifications 9

R
Rapport 45
Rate of perceived exertion 88
Register of exercise professionals 12
Relative strength 58
Resistance training 105
Reversibility 80
Risk assessment 35
Rockport 56

S
Salt 147
Session structure 129
Scoliosis 69
Screening 70
Single set training 107

SMART goals 99
Sports drinks
Split routine 134
Sports drinks 146
Stage of change 45
Step test 56
Stress 75
Stretching 124
Static stretching 124
Studio instructor 9
Supersets 108

T
Talk test 90
Tri-sets 109

U
Unique selling point 25

V
Vitamins 140,141
Volunteering 17

W
Waist to hip ratio 61
Water 145

Printed in Great Britain
by Amazon